Fantastic Water Workouts

SECOND EDITION

MaryBeth Pappas Baun

Human Kinetics

Library of Congress Cataloging-in-Publication Data

Gaines, MaryBeth Pappas, 1957-
Fantastic water workouts / MaryBeth Pappas Baun. -- 2nd ed.
  p. cm.
Includes index.
ISBN-13: 978-0-7360-6808-6 (soft cover)
ISBN-10: 0-7360-6808-2 (soft cover)
1. Aquatic exercises. I. Title.
GV838.53.E94G35 2008
613.7'16--dc22
                2007036103
ISBN-10: 0-7360-6808-2
ISBN-13: 978-0-7360-6808-6

This publication is written and published to provide accurate and authoritative information relevant to the subject matter presented. It is published and sold with the understanding that the author and publisher are not engaged in rendering legal, medical, or other professional services by reason of their authorship or publication of this work. If medical or other expert assistance is required, the services of a competent professional person should be sought.

The Web addresses cited in this text were current as of October 1, 2007, unless otherwise noted.

Acquisitions Editor: Laurel Plotzke; **Developmental Editor:** Kevin Matz; **Assistant Editor:** Laura Koritz; **Copyeditor:** Susan Campanini; **Proofreader:** Bethany J. Bentley; **Indexer:** Craig Brown; **Permission Manager:** Carly Breeding; **Graphic Designer:** Nancy Rasmus; **Cover Designer:** Keith Blomberg; **Photographer (cover):** Will Funk; **Photographer (interior):** James Wiseman; **Visual Production Assistant:** Joyce Brumfield; **Photo Office Assistant:** Jason Allen; **Art Manager:** Kelly Hendren; **Associate Art Manager:** Al Wilborn; **Illustrator:** Dianna Porter; **Printer:** United Graphics

Yoga Booty Ballet on pages 194-202 adapted by permission of Gillian Marloth Clark and Teigh McDonough. Water Yoga on pages 182-187 and Tai Chi on pages 171-178 adapted by permission of Carol Argo.

We thank the Memorial Hermann Wellness Center in Houston, Texas, for assistance in providing the location for the photo shoot for this book.

Human Kinetics books are available at special discounts for bulk purchase. Special editions or book excerpts can also be created to specification. For details, contact the Special Sales Manager at Human Kinetics.

Printed in the United States of America   10 9 8 7 6 5 4 3 2 1

Human Kinetics
Web site: www.HumanKinetics.com

United States: Human Kinetics
P.O. Box 5076
Champaign, IL 61825-5076
800-747-4457
e-mail: humank@hkusa.com

Canada: Human Kinetics
475 Devonshire Road Unit 100
Windsor, ON N8Y 2L5
800-465-7301 (in Canada only)
e-mail: orders@hkcanada.com

Europe: Human Kinetics
107 Bradford Road, Stanningley
Leeds LS28 6AT, United Kingdom
+44 (0) 113 255 5665
e-mail: hk@hkeurope.com

Australia: Human Kinetics
57A Price Avenue
Lower Mitcham, South Australia 5062
08 8372 0999
e-mail: info@hkaustralia.com

New Zealand: Human Kinetics
Division of Sports Distributors NZ Ltd.
P.O. Box 300 226 Albany
North Shore City, Auckland
0064 9 448 1207
e-mail: info@humankinetics.co.nz

Dedicated to my husband, William Boyd Baun, in deep gratitude for his love, inspiration, and support.

CONTENTS

Water exercise has rapidly increased in popularity. People from all walks of life—fitness enthusiasts; athletes of all stripes, professional, elite, and recreational; people with health issues or injuries; older adults; and people who just want to have fun—have discovered that something special happens when you work out in water: It works! All over the world, individuals and groups have found that water workouts suit their fitness needs and fit their lifestyle. Water workouts have earned recognition for the unique combination of advantages they offer: a total body workout that moves your body through functional ranges of motion that build core strength against multidirectional resistance, while minimizing joint stress and reducing risk of injury, in a comfortable environment that keeps you cool.

According to the *Fitness Management Journal* (2004), more than 6 million Americans participate in water exercise. Over the past decade, the research community has led the charge, with study after study demonstrating the benefits of water-based exercise. Why has water fitness gained so much attention? The Surgeon General recommends 30 minutes or more of moderate physical activity on most days for good health. But people find it difficult to make that a habit. The majority do not currently engage in regular physical activity. Of those who start an exercise program, 70 percent drop out within one year. Many reasons lead to dropout, and most people stop because they have chosen an activity that doesn't suit them properly. They may find it painful or boring, or it just doesn't fit with their interests, schedule, or social needs. Water provides an environment that makes it possible to overcome all of these obstacles.

The properties of water provide a unique environment for people of all abilities to get a better workout in less time. These properties include buoyancy, multidirectional resistance (hydrostatic pressure), higher resistance via viscosity, and enhanced cooling. Water lends itself to a well-balanced workout that improves all major components of physical fitness: aerobic endurance, muscular strength and endurance, flexibility, and posture and body composition. It also improves coordination, agility, stability, mobility, and balance, which are critical not only for athletes, but also for day-to-day successful living and for those who want to stay mobile in the later years of life. This is especially important in U.S. society, where the number of older adults, thanks to the Baby Boomer generation, is predicted to double in the first thirty years of the twenty-first century. Why is mobility so important? Because adequate mobility equals greater independence and better health and well-being.

The aquatic techniques used in water workouts produce overall, total-body fitness that rivals the results of many other forms of exercise. Water exercisers achieve greater involvement of the entire body than is possible during land-based aerobic activities, such as cycling or jogging, that focus on specific repetitive actions. Perhaps most important, water motivates people to exercise because it is stimulating and fun. Water makes working out a pleasurable, comfortable, refreshing, and invigorating experience.

For more than a decade, researchers who study exercise physiology and health have expanded the body of evidence that supports what water exercise enthusiasts have reported. The documentation is in, the evidence is clear, and water workout fans have the evidence for their claims: Water workouts produce health and fitness benefits while burning more calories in less time, and they cause less discomfort and provide better protection from injuries. Not surprisingly, people enjoy their workouts more and stick with them longer, thereby increasing the opportunity to make physical activity a regular part of their lives.

Why does water fitness work?

- Water adds more resistance, 12 to 14 percent more than when you exercise on land. Every move you make in water increases resistance for your muscles, which improves strength and can help increase your metabolism, or the rate at which you burn calories, even at rest.

- Water provides multidirectional resistance. Your muscles typically work in pairs, and the resistance of water allows you to work opposing muscle groups in balance, without having to reposition yourself and repeat the exercise as you would on land to achieve similar results. And, the multidirectional resistance creates an environment ideal for functional conditioning—the kind that makes your body work better as a unified linkage system.

- Water acts as a cushion for your body. According to the Aquatic Exercise Association, your body, when immersed up to the chest, bears approximately 25 to 30 percent of your total body weight. Immersed to the waist, it bears 50 percent. This buoyancy allows many people to do movements that might otherwise be difficult on land, and creates a shock-absorbing crosstraining environment that prevents injuries for everyone.

- Water regulates your temperature, protecting you from overheating. You don't feel hot or sweaty, so you are more comfortable during your workout.

Researchers concur that there are many benefits to working out in the water:

- Water workouts help you improve strength and flexibility in less time.

- Exercising in the water allows you to improve or maintain your body weight and body composition (ratio of lean to fatty tissue).

- Aqua aerobics meet ACSM (American College of Sports Medicine) fitness guidelines for building cardiorespiratory endurance.

- Water helps protect you from bone loss that can lead to osteoporosis.

- Working out in water can rehabilitate or prevent injury to your muscles. (For example, water decreases swelling and offsets the pooling of blood in your extremities.)

- Water exercise provides social benefits for those who participate in group classes.

- Working out in the water fosters a positive attitude, feelings of well-being, and relief from stress and anxiety.

There is extensive research showing the benefits of water fitness participation for the following health challenges:

- Arthritis
- Multiple sclerosis
- Back pain, knee pain, rehabilitation
- Diabetes
- Fibromyalgia
- Prenatal and postnatal conditions
- Cardiac conditions

The first edition of *Fantastic Water Workouts* motivated tens of thousands of people worldwide to become involved in water workouts. This second edition builds on the first and offers easy-to-read, easy-to-follow movement instructions paired with over- and underwater photos that make them simple to use. It shares with you what you need in order to become successful with water workouts, either as a participant or an instructor. You gain concise, complete information on how to get the best results for your goals and the kind of information you need to enhance your skills and abilities and address special concerns. This edition includes diverse styles, equipment, and moves that have generated new excitement in the world of water workouts and tips about the best ways to engage your core so that you are strong functionally as well as sleek and fit in appearance. Many agree that the best part of the second edition is the toned, sleek body that you can achieve with the new core strength and posture-building moves for sculpting your abdomen, torso, hips, and buttocks. The power of these moves is in their ability to enhance postural alignment and help prevent and improve pain in your back, neck, shoulders, and knees. The beauty of these moves is that they make you look better in and out of your clothes. The wisdom is that they help you function more strongly in daily activities while enhancing your overall health and well-being.

Times have changed: Since the early 1990s, there has been tremendous growth in the number of pools available to people who want to work out in the water. Year-round pool access is not a problem in most areas. People are trying a new and wider range of diverse activities to start and maintain their interest in staying physically active—Yoga, Tai Chi, Pilates, kickboxing, line dancing, ballet, hip-hop, Spinning—and they are taking those activities into the water. New gear makes water workouts more comfortable: better flotation belts and vests, warmer suits, swimsuits that don't ride up, more supportive aqua shoes. New water tools and toys make being in the water more fun and more effective, adding innovative ways to increase resistance, provide more comfortable flotation, use a bike or treadmill in the water, or even run on top of the water at the beach or on a river.

When I wrote the first edition of *Fantastic Water Workouts* in the early 1990s, aqua therapy was something to think about as an alternative. Now it is accepted as the right thing to do; in many cases, it is considered best practice for (1) increasing fitness and athletic performance without generating trauma or damage, (2) treating pain, illness, and injury, and (3) providing a cross-training workout that's just plain fun.

I have included all of these developments in this new edition. In the second edition of *Fantastic Water Workouts*, step-by-step illustrated instructions guide you from the first simple-to-learn water workout to the well-rounded basic water workout, all the way to the advanced and intensified moves of *aqua power* (push-off moves that tone your hips and buttocks while you build strength and aerobic intensity) and *plyometrics* (jump-training techniques that raise aerobic intensity, challenge your muscles, and improve your performance). Advanced Fantastic Water Workout moves that apply these principles and build core strength include Pilates (concentrated strength and flexibility methods that focus on the powerhouse of the abs and buttocks), kickboxing (uses the upper body for a variety of punches and lower body for kicks), and Yoga Booty Ballet (combines yoga, dance, and body sculpting). Core strength—meaning firm, functionally strong, and flexible torso, neck, and lower-body muscles—is key to wellness and musculoskeletal health. A sequence of abdominal workout techniques shows you how to produce sleek, strong abdominals using the unique, intensifying yet gentle properties of water. A series of strengthening moves for the back and neck challenge postural muscles to improve stability to prepare you for whatever life throws your way.

People with specific goals can find tailored sequences and instructions to guide them through Tone Up and Weight Loss; the Pregnancy Workout; Water Workouts for back, neck, or knee pain; the Water Workout for Older Adults; the Cardiac Recovery Workout; the Arthritis Workout; and programs and tips for people with fibromyalgia, multiple sclerosis, plantar fasciitis, or diabetes.

This book describes how water exercise can improve your fitness enjoyably and safely. It gives you the information you need to improve your fitness level gradually without the aches, pains, injuries, and frustrations that are sometimes associated with a fitness program. Chapter 2, Preparing for Water Workouts, gets you started with your water workouts by helping you prepare the best environment and informing you about how to equip yourself with a variety of water tools, equipment, and shoes to enhance your water exercise experience.

Next are descriptions of water workouts for flexibility, aerobics, and muscle strengthening and toning and explanations of the importance of warm-up and cool-down exercises. There are easy-to-follow instructions, photographs, and objectives for 135 exercises in this book. Instructions on tailored sequencing help you devise routines that are fun, safe, and specific to your objectives.

In chapters 7 through 10, you'll learn how to personalize a workout for your goals and needs. If you want to intensify your workouts or add some new excitement, chapter 7, Intensifying Workouts, takes you through challenging power and plyometrics workouts. In chapter 8, Creating a Personal Water Workout, you learn about your particular body type and how it affects your workout choices. Chapter 8 also defines Tone Up and Weight Loss approaches and explains the methods and value of incorporating variations into your water workouts. Chapter 9, Adding Splash to Workouts, is full of sizzling new techniques, such as Water Yoga, Water Pilates, Water Kickboxing, Water Hip-Hop, Water Country Line Dancing, and Water Yoga Booty Ballet™. If you want to use your workouts to help with specific health concerns, you'll discover how to set reachable goals and choose the right exercises for your situation in chapter 10, Specializing Workouts for Special Needs. The second edition of *Fantastic Water Workouts* gets you started right and keeps you going with many ways to keep your water workouts fun, effective, and exciting!

In the late 1980s, when water exercise was just beginning its gradual climb to popularity, I was very active physically. In addition to teaching aerobics 8 to 10 times a week, running, and playing tennis and wallyball, I also loved hiking, canoeing, and biking. What I did not realize was that my body was taking a pounding. My back, knees, and feet did not put up with this unin-tentionally abusive physical lifestyle for long, but I wasn't about to give up, so "cross-training" became a necessity. Water exercise became my salvation, and I wanted to share my newfound joy. I found water workouts more fun than any other activity I was involved in. Best of all, as a fitness instructor and wellness coach, I am committed to making physical activity accessible to everyone: Water workouts have the qualities to bridge the gap for almost everyone, by making physical activity possible and more effective for all kinds of people of all ages. This book is written as a guide that brings together the many lessons I have learned about water workouts over the years from my own body; from my clients and their experiences; from sports medicine physicians, aquatic certification leaders, water exercise divas, physical therapists, scientific researchers; and from the commercial world of aqua aerobics. I hope that this book—and the water exercise it gets you hooked on—bring you as much joy as it has me. And I hope to meet you in the pool someday!

So, what are you waiting for? Let's dive in!

CHAPTER 1

Improving Fitness With Water Exercises

Exercise on a regular basis, including water workouts, enhances your overall health and well-being. Water exercise boosts your ability to achieve these results in greater comfort and with the joy and exhilaration that you can experience in an aquatic environment. Anyone who wants to build better fitness and protect his or her health can reap the rewards that water exercise has to offer. People whose goals include building cardiorespiratory endurance, improving strength and flexibility, improving or maintaining body weight and composition, or rehabilitating or preventing injuries can benefit from water exercise. Highly fit individuals delight in the opportunity to gain high-intensity cross-training by working out in the low-impact, high-resistance environment of water. Athletes improve performance while minimizing risks. People who want to manage their weight enjoy the chance to burn more calories in less time, with less risk of injury to the joints and the back. Fitness enthusiasts enjoy the fun of water workouts while getting functional training that most land-based programs, with or without equipment, can't match for quick and efficient results. Pregnant women who need the buoyancy and cooling effects of water find the aquatic environment relieving and stimulating. People who are managing or preventing special conditions—such as heart disease, back pain, diabetes, fibromyalgia, arthritis, injuries, or just about any movement limitation—become liberated by the qualities of exercise in water for fitness and rehabilitation. Everyone who wants to add splash to a dry routine will find that water workouts have multiple benefits for anyone interested in movement for fitness and health.

Exercise for fitness can become more fun, effective, interesting, motivating, and healing when you add the comfort and invigorating dynamics of water. When you get used to the novel feeling of moving around in the aquatic

1

environment, you'll have a sense of fitness mastery and movement freedom in water exercise that you can't easily get on land.

Millions of individuals use water workouts to gain these advantages:

- Heart, lungs, and circulatory system work more efficiently.
- Energy increases.
- Metabolism speeds up.
- Sleep improves (even more so when you include stretching).
- Weight control and body composition improvement become easier to manage.
- Negative stress and tension get released.
- Cholesterol and blood pressure levels can be improved.
- Depression and anxiety can lessen.
- Comfort during pregnancy can be enhanced.
- Diabetes management can improve and need for medications can be reduced.
- Risk of cancer can be lowered.
- Attitude and self-confidence benefit.

Although water workouts are ideal for the average person for a variety of reasons, the unique benefits of water exercise have also influenced professional and elite athletes to use water workouts to improve performance, speed recovery from injury, and enhance physical conditioning. Outstanding professional athletes, including NBA forward Kevin McHale, NFL quarterback Joe Montana, skating champions Nancy Kerrigan and Paul Wylie, and football and baseball hero Bo Jackson, have led the charge to using water exercise for improving health and fitness. Discovery that water exercise shortens recovery time led quickly to the realization that fitness and performance could also be greatly enhanced with the appropriate water workout techniques.

One athlete who demonstrated the power of water is Nancy Kerrigan, who was seriously injured less than two months before skating to an Olympic silver medal in 1994. How did she do it? Water aerobics rehabilitated her knee and provided phenomenal aerobic workouts, sending her quickly on her way to victory. Until the mid-1980s, the idea of a professional athlete using aquatics for anything more than injury rehabilitation was considered unusual. Today, athletes from many sport disciplines incorporate aquatic training into their workout regimen to enhance fitness and peak performance. Members of the Chicago Bulls, Cleveland Cavaliers, Miami Dolphins, San Francisco 49ers, Minnesota Vikings, and boxing star Evander Holyfield all use aquatic training on a regular basis.

Benefits of Water Workouts

People who want to maximize results and minimize risk of injury have been incorporating the benefits of water workouts more than ever before. Sports medicine research has fueled this trend. Deep-water running with flotation cuts down on the compression of the spine compared to running on land, and so it reduces spinal shrinkage. This effect of "unloading" the pressure on the spine is important, because 80 percent of people experience debilitating back pain at one time or another and compression of the vertebrae and discs is a major cause.

Medical research has uncovered additional reasons to make water exercise a habit. Aquatic exercise results in better total cholesterol levels, as well as improvements in aerobic fitness, weight, strength, flexibility, and agility. A single experience of participating in water exercise was shown to reduce anxiety. In a study of women of childbearing age, aquatic exercise resulted in improved pregnancy outcomes, fewer hospitalizations, delivery of healthier babies, and reduced illness in mothers and babies after delivery.

Water exercise provides an ideal and safe form of workout for just about everyone. By exercising in water, you can increase the blood supply to your muscles, burn more stored nutrients (calories) by producing more energy for movement, increase your body's use of oxygen, and decrease your blood pressure. By reducing stress on muscles, bones, tendons, and ligaments, some people who can't exercise comfortably on land find that they can exercise in water. Even people with conditions that may interfere with exercise—such as arthritis, back pain, heart disease, fibromyalgia, obesity, multiple sclerosis, or pregnancy—can enjoy the benefits of exercising in water. These are some of the main reasons for anyone to take advantage of water exercise:

- Reduce stress on your joints, bones, and muscles.
- Achieve speedy, effective toning through water resistance.
- Increase your exercise work load and burn more calories in less time.
- Stay cooler, even when you are exercising hard.
- Experience the ideal combination of fun, effective training, and comfort.

Reduces Joint, Bone, and Muscle Stress

Because of the buoyancy of water, your perceived body weight can be as much as 90 percent less in water than your actual body weight on land (the percentage varies depending on the water depth). So weight-bearing impact shock is minimal in water, particularly compared to land-based running or aerobic dance. With flotation devices, you can eliminate impact completely. Exercise in water is also less apt to lead to the muscle soreness that most people experience when they start or intensify an exercise program on land.

Impact shock is one of the most common culprits in muscle soreness and joint pain after exercise. The buoyancy of water takes the pressure off your joint capsule, which, in combination with the warmth of the water, increases your ability to move comfortably and with greater flexibility. Your risk of joint pain is reduced and existing joint pain can be relieved while you are exercising appropriately in water.

Weight training in water also minimizes the possibility of muscle, bone, and joint injuries because water provides resistance to your body in multiple directions. Compare working with weights or resistance on land and in water: On land, you can become injured if you lift too heavy a weight and do not have adequate strength to lower it safely; you are resisting the forces of gravity and fighting the weight's downward pressure. In water, which is more dense than air, you meet resistance in both directions as you move your body; you meet the viscosity of water in all directions. This phenomenon also develops balanced muscle strength (which helps prevent injury) by working the muscles on both sides of your joints during each repetition of the same exercise.

Tones Through Water Resistance

As an exercise environment, water is more dense than air. Therefore, by harnessing the resistive power of water, you can speed up your conditioning and enhance your toning results. Pushing or pulling your limbs through water approximates the use of muscle power required for weight training without the discomfort. In fact, when you use the appropriate equipment for water-resistance training, water workouts can produce results comparable to those achieved in land-based weight training programs designed to enhance muscle strength and tone.

Because water provides resistance in multiple directions whereas gravity (on land) is unidirectional in force, exercising in water lets you accomplish just as much as on land, but in less time. On land, to work two opposing muscle groups (muscles on two sides of a joint that must be worked evenly to maintain muscle balance, stabilize joints, and prevent injury, such as the front and the back of your thighs or your chest and upper back), you must change your position and repeat the exercise. But in water, the resistance allows you to work two opposing muscle groups with each repetition. For example, a biceps curl (bending your elbow and bringing your palm upward) works the front of your upper arm (biceps), on land or in the water. But in water, the action of returning to a straight arm position meets the resistance of the water and works the back of your upper arm (triceps) as well. Because working two opposing muscle groups simultaneously develops muscle tone more efficiently, you build muscle faster by working in water than by working on land.

Other important relationships include your abdominal muscles and lower back, your hip flexors (used in the Knee Lift) and your buttocks and hamstrings, your outer and inner thighs, and your shins and calves. To help you balance your muscle work, each exercise, stretch, and movement illustrated in this book identifies the muscles being worked or stretched. Use this information when planning your balanced water workout.

Increases Workload and Burns Calories

Because it takes more muscle energy to push your body through water than through air, walking in thigh-deep water or in deep water with an exercise flotation device can give you more than double the workload of walking on land. Your energy utilization system works harder, too. You can burn up to 525 calories per hour by water walking compared with 240 calories on land, without getting hot and with less risk of injury. For variety and overall improved fitness results, walk forward, backward, and sideways, with short steps, long steps, average steps, steps touches, or step kicks. These movement variations and changes of direction can prevent muscle overuse injury and increase your workload.

Prevents Overheating

A common reason people avoid exercise is that they experience discomfort with increased physical activity. Water workouts solve the comfort problem. Besides reducing impact and joint stress, they won't leave you sweaty. Your body transmits exercise heat to water more easily than to air, to keep you cool and comfortable.

Combines Fun, Training, and Comfort

Water invigorates you. Splashing around in a swimming pool is playful; it makes people smile, perhaps because exercise can be more pleasant in water. Calisthenics become more interesting, more comfortable, and a lot more fun. If you prefer comfort over strain, the cooling effects and supportive buoyancy of water make exercise and stretches feel deceptively easy. Yet experienced fitness devotees appreciate the high resistance of water, which enhances toning, strength building, and calorie burning.

Your likelihood of success in establishing any new exercise habit rests firmly on the degree of pleasure you get from that activity. Human behavior studies by Ferris and Henderson indicate that, to get someone involved in a particular form of exercise over the long term, "the program must be fun, satisfying, or enjoyable." Those who try water exercise enjoy moving in the aquatic environment.

Building a Better Body

"Fitness" consists of several major components that affect your body strength, tone, endurance, mobility, and resistance to illness and injury: flexibility, muscular strength and endurance, body composition, and cardiorespiratory or aerobic endurance. Sport physiologists also identify several motor skills that are also considered fitness components: speed, power (strength and speed in one explosive action), agility (ability to change body position), coordination (ability to integrate separate motor activities into one smooth motion), reaction time, and balance (ability to maintain equilibrium). Water exercise programs provide many opportunities to move through exercises that enhance each major fitness component and a multitude of motor skills.

You make progress in all of the fitness categories when you exercise regularly using the well-rounded Basic Water Workout on page 42 in chapter 3, Understanding the Phases of a Water Workout. The specific kind of training you emphasize determines which fitness components improve most. Follow a program that emphasizes the conditioning techniques that help you achieve your personal fitness objectives. The categories that follow provide information to help you choose what to emphasize during your workouts to enhance your health and fitness.

Flexibility

Flexibility is the ability of your joints to move through a full range of motion. Range of motion refers to the degree to which there is movement around a joint. Pain-free posture and healthy, pain-free mobility of your musculoskeletal system require that you maintain an adequate range of motion at all of your joints. People who avoid stretching or who stretch incorrectly frequently experience joint and muscle injuries that result from inadequate flexibility or joint stress. Range of motion activities, especially in warm water, can be particularly beneficial for people with arthritis, injuries, and joint or back pain.

Muscle Strength and Endurance

Muscle strength is measured by the amount of force you can exert in a single effort through the full range of motion. *Muscle endurance* is your ability to exert a moderate amount of force through a full range of motion over an extended period before the onset of fatigue.

Developing and maintaining good muscle strength throughout your lifetime has been shown to improve physical independence and mobility dramatically in the later years of life. If you want to improve your muscle strength, increase your resistance. To emphasize muscle endurance over strength, lower the amount of resistance and increase the number of repetitions. But avoid high levels of resistance if you have symptoms or risk of illness or injury.

Body Composition

Body composition is the proportion of lean body mass to fatty body mass in your body. Lean body mass includes bone, muscle, tendons, nerves, and ligaments. Aerobic activities can train your body to be a better fat burner; reducing excess body fat can reduce your risk of heart disease or cancer. Muscle strength and endurance activities will improve lean body mass and help to ensure long-term weight control. However, people today strive, often unsuccessfully, to emulate the unrealistic slender ideal portrayed by movie stars and supermodels. The proliferation of slender role models has helped create an unhealthy craze of extreme dieting and exercise, rampant eating disorders, and exaggerated exercise expectations among both men and women who believe that everyone can and should be slim. Exercise and proper diet can indeed cause an individual to lose weight, but several research studies indicate that it is unrealistic to assume that everyone can develop a thin figure. In fact, thinner is not necessarily healthier for men or women, and studies of mortality rates show similar risk levels for a broad range of body compositions. In other words, people vary widely and a wide range of body compositions are associated with good health. Weight loss intervention does not significantly decrease health risk unless your initial body fat ratio exceeds 27 percent. Instead of focusing on "being thin," aspire to get and stay fit, and enjoy the journey and the process of making water exercise a regular part of your life.

If you are curious about your own body composition, visit a local health club or sports medicine clinic to have it measured once or twice a year. There is no completely infallible way to measure body composition, so have the same person do the measurement each time and use the same techniques to make sure you are making an even comparison from one measurement to the next.

MYTHS AND MISCONCEPTIONS

Myth: You can whittle down your waistline by performing sit-ups or shrink your thighs with leg lifts.

FALSE There is no such thing as spot reducing. It's true that you can firm and strengthen soft muscles by performing abdominal exercises and leg lifts. But to lose inches, you must perform aerobic exercise regularly, such as 20 minutes or more of brisk walking three to five times a week. Regular aerobic exercise burns off stored fat overall. Creating more toned (firm and strong) muscles through resistance exercises helps you keep the fat off by enhancing your metabolic rate (you burn more calories even at rest). The beauty of water exercise is that you burn calories aerobically while at the same time toning your muscles by pushing through the resistance of water.

Cardiorespiratory and Aerobic Endurance

Aerobic fitness is also called *cardiorespiratory endurance* because it involves the ability of your heart, lungs, and circulatory system to supply oxygen to your muscles during exercise. Aerobic activity stimulates your body's ability to sustain an activity within the aerobic training zone for an extended period. Regular, moderate aerobic exercise enhances stress management, improves sleep, assists weight control, increases fat burning, helps control appetite, improves energy levels, and reduces the incidence of heart disease and other ailments.

Finding the Target Zone

There is an optimal level of exercise intensity, called the *target zone*, that is required to improve your cardiorespiratory fitness. If you exercise below your target zone, you don't challenge your body sufficiently to improve aerobic endurance. By exercising above your target zone, you put excessive stress on your system and increase your potential for injury, illness, low energy, and exhaustion, without gaining more fitness.

For an exercise to be aerobic and strengthen the cardiorespiratory system, it must train your body to do a better job of delivering oxygen to your performing muscles. When you exercise above your target zone, your body must turn to the anaerobic (without oxygen) energy system. This system is designed to work for only short periods, which explains why fatigue is the end result of exercise beyond the intensity of your target zone.

A simple way to check your aerobic intensity is to use the "Talk Test." If you can still speak while exercising but are breathing a bit more heavily, you are working at an aerobic level, within your target zone.

Measuring Intensity With Heart Rate

You can find out whether or not you are exercising at the optimal intensity during an aerobic or cardiorespiratory activity by monitoring your heart rate. A little practice makes it easy to find your pulse and count the beats. Practice when you are sitting still and when you are moving.

One way to monitor your heart rate is to use your radial artery: Locate the pulse on your wrist with the index and middle fingers of your dominant hand (right, if you are right-handed; left, if you are left-handed). Gently place your fingers against the thumb side of your wrist (see figure 1.1a). Your thumb is not used because it has a pulse of its own that can be misleading in determining your heart rate.

A second way to monitor your heart rate is by using your carotid artery, below your jaw: Place the tip of your thumb in the middle of your chin. Move your palm toward your jaw, and place your index and middle fingers at the hollow of your neck just below the jawbone. Keep your head up straight and lightly adjust the position of your fingers until you can feel your pulse (see figure 1.1b). Press *lightly* to avoid cutting off your circulation. If you press too hard, you slow your heartbeat and you could become dizzy or faint.

Taking Your Resting Heart Rate   Take your resting heart rate after you have been sitting quietly for 15 minutes or, better yet, when you first wake up in the morning (after waking naturally or staying still in bed for a few minutes

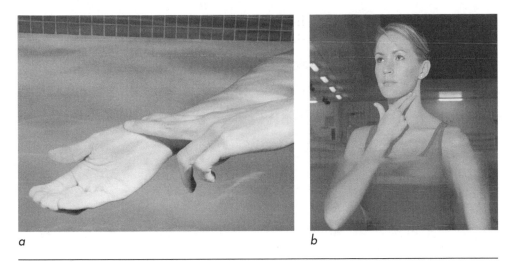

a   b

Figure 1.1   Monitoring heart rate using *(a)* the radial artery and *(b)* the carotid artery.

after waking by clock alarm) and before getting out of bed. Find your pulse at your radial artery at the wrist or at your carotid artery at the neck and count for 15 seconds while watching a clock. Multiply the result by 4 to get the number of beats per minute.

Your resting heart rate count can give you a general idea of your cardio-respiratory fitness. If your total beats per minute are less than 60, you are probably aerobically fit and can maintain your current level of activity. If your count is more than 60, you may need to increase your level or frequency of aerobic exercise gradually. There are many exceptions to this rule of thumb, including for people who take antihypertensive drugs or have other medical conditions that affect their resting heart rate.

Finding Your Working Heart Rate   Monitor your heart rate during the first part of your aerobic activity and again just after the peak of training intensity. A slow warm-up is important to prepare your body gradually for the vigorous work you are planning to give your cardiovascular system. During this time, your heart rate should build toward the low end of your target range.

To monitor your working heart rate, find your pulse and watch a clock with a digital display or a sweep-second hand. Count the number of heartbeats for 6 seconds and multiply by 10. This gives you your heartbeat rate per minute. Refer to table 1.1 to determine the number of beats per minute that correspond to your desired working heart rate.

If your heart rate is less than your target rate during aerobic conditioning, take longer steps (within what is both comfortable and controllable), lift your knees higher, use stronger arm movements, or add water resistance equipment. If your heart rate is more than your target, move less vigorously, use smaller steps, keep your arm movements small, or reduce resistance.

Table 1.1 Target Zone Working Heart Rate Range for Water Exercise

Age	HEARTBEATS PER MINUTE		
	60	70	80
	(% OF AGE-PREDICTED MAXIMUM HEART RATE)		
10	110	135	155
15	110	130	150
20	105	125	145
25	100	120	140
30	100	120	135
35	95	115	135
40	95	110	130
45	90	110	125
50	85	105	120
55	85	100	115
60	80	95	115
65	80	95	110
70+	75	90	105

The chart above indicates aquatic aerobic targets. Heart rates in water are lower than on land, even though the people exercising are working out at the same level of oxygen consumption. Oxygen consumption levels indicate the actual intensity and energy output of an exercise.

Measuring Intensity by How You Feel: Rate of Perceived Exertion (RPE)

Personal perceptions of effort are closely related to actual workload, heart rate, oxygen consumption, and even lactic acid (an exercise by-product) and hormones. Therefore, your subjective estimate of work intensity provides an accurate estimate of the level of intensity and your body's internal responses to exercise. Because you are able to judge your effort accurately, it is important to "listen to yourself" during exercise. If the exercise feels too intense, it probably is. Monitor how your heart, lungs, and circulatory system feel during aerobic exercise. Avoid including perceptions of physical difficulty based on whether it is hard or easy to coordinate, maneuver, or maintain your balance or whether the water is making your body more comfortable than on land. These perceptions do not relate to your aerobic intensity. The perception of exertion is based mainly on the fatigue of your muscles and the feeling of breathlessness.

The perceived exertion rate scale (table 1.2) allows you to monitor your exertion easily. As illustrated, a 9 corresponds to very light exercise. For a normal, healthy person, this is like walking slowly for some minutes. A 13 is "somewhat hard" exercise, but still feels OK to continue. A 17 is very strenuous and a healthy person can go on but it's a struggle and the person feels very heavy and is tired. A 19 is extremely strenuous and for most people is the most strenuous exercise they have experienced. Between 10 and 16 a person's heart rate would be at about 60-80% of his or her target heart rate.

Most people should exercise within the range of "somewhat hard" to "hard" to achieve aerobic fitness. For instance, when you measure your intensity using the heart rate monitoring system, the exercise feels "somewhat hard" when you exercise at a target heart rate of about 70 percent of your age-predicted maximum heart rate. "Somewhat hard" corresponds to a moderate level of aerobic exertion.

Therefore, you can use your sense of difficulty to guide your exertion. One of the advantages of using this method is that your perception of exertion signals you to slow your pace to a more prudent level if high temperatures cause your heart rate to rise. The second benefit of using perceived exertion is that it eliminates the need to monitor your heart rate while the challenging environment of lapping water interferes with your ability to find your pulse.

Table 1.2 The Borg RPE Scale for Perceived Exertion

6	No exertion at all
7	Extremely light
8	
9	Very light
10	
11	Light
12	
13	Somewhat hard
14	
15	Hard (heavy)
16	
17	Very hard
18	
19	Extremely hard
20	Maximal exertion

Reprinted, by permission, from G. Borg, 1988, "Borg's perceived exertion and pain scales" (Champaign, IL: Human Kinetics), 47. © Gunnar Borg, 1970, 1985, 1994, 1998

Effects of Water on Heart Rate

Because of the effects of water on the physiology of the cardiovascular system, physiologists recommend targeting 10 to 20 beats less in water compared to land. According to researchers this difference is attributable to two factors: Exercise in water temperatures from 77 to 85 degrees Fahrenheit (25 to 29 degrees Celsius) produces a lower heart rate response, and water pressure on the body helps circulate the blood.

The hydrostatic pressure of water shifts blood volume away from the limbs and toward the chest, heart, and lungs. This shift increases central venous pressure, stroke volume, and cardiac output, which leads to a decrease in the heart rate compared to working at the same level of oxygen consumption on land. In other words, the pressure of the water helps the heart circulate blood by aiding the veins in returning blood flow back to the heart. This assistance to the heart contributes to lower blood pressure and heart rates during deep-water exercise versus similar exertions on land.

This difference is partly because water assists and improves the blood flow to the heart. Water dissipates heat more effectively than air, and the body compensates by constricting the blood vessels in the limbs. This in turn increases blood flow to the heart (lowering heart rate) and also increases the amount of blood output with each heartbeat. Scientists also found that exercise in water results in the same cardiac output (amount of blood discharged by the heart per minute) per liter of oxygen consumed as on land. In other words, even though the heart rate may be lower in water for a similar exercise on land, the body is delivering more oxygenated blood to the working muscles per beat. Therefore, the body is working as hard to deliver the same amount of oxygen as on land, even though the measured heart rate is about 10 beats lower for vertical exercise and 17 beats lower for horizontal exercise in water. Water exercisers can gain the same aerobic exercise benefits as they would on land. Researchers at Adelphi University found that, even though water-based heart rates were 13 percent lower than land-based counts, the water exercisers achieved the same benefits as their land-based counterparts.

Preferred Exertion

Preferred exertion is the concept that each of us seems to require a certain level of exertion in a workout to be satisfied. If the exertion is too little or too great, satisfaction is diminished. Training or exercising regularly increases the amount of exertion preferred, and inactivity lowers it.

People who have been involved in competitive sports often prefer a high level of exertion. Also a misconception among many athletes is that exercise has to hurt to be good. It does not. And when they resume activity after a long break, they overdo it, and end up with a lot of soreness. This also creates a potential for injury.

Caution

Fitness cannot be stored in your body. If you must miss several workouts because of illness or scheduling conflicts, work at a lower level when you return to exercise until you have recovered your original state of fitness.

Body Movement in Water

The unique characteristics of water make it an excellent medium for multiple exercise goals and for every type of exerciser. The term *hydrodynamics* refers to the physical principles associated with moving your body in water. By understanding how best to use those principles, you can devise safe and effective routines for water exercise and can more readily perform the specific exercises illustrated in the chapters that follow. Several specific hydrodynamic principles explain the various ways that water affects your body. Use these descriptions of hydrodynamics to get started, enhance your water exercise program, and guide your progression.

Buoyancy

The less dense an object is, the more it is inclined to float. Humans are less dense than water and therefore are apt to float. Of course, every person has a different propensity to float, based on the percentage of fat to bone and lean muscle and the amount of air the lungs can hold. Therefore, some people experience more exaggerated effects of buoyancy than others. Greater buoyancy may reduce impact shock, but it may also make it more difficult to control movements and posture in water.

The buoyancy that water produces can enhance your muscle workout and decrease the harmful effects of impact shock. The force that buoyancy generates can add either assistance or resistance to movements performed under-water. Buoyancy makes it easier to move toward the surface of the water and harder to move away from the surface.

The water you displace when you enter the water creates buoyancy and produces the nonweight-bearing aspect of exercising in water that makes jumping and running more comfortable. Buoyancy neutralizes gravity and diminishes the harmful stress of impact on your body. Buoyancy and the equalized pressure of water around a joint also reduce the pressure of gravity on your joint capsule, working with the warmth of the water to create a more pain-free environment for increasing range of motion in stiff joints. You can jump higher, leap farther, run or walk longer, and push harder in water because of the comfortable, protective environment that it creates.

Buoyancy can also alter your posture. People who have greater buoyancy, especially originating in the chest and buttocks, may be inclined to arch at the lower back, causing an increased *lordotic curve*. This curve at the base of your spine can put stress on your lower back if your abdominals and buttocks are not held in firmly to maintain a healthy posture. To protect your lower back and to compensate for the tendency to arch inwardly at the lower back, adopt the pelvic "braced neutral position" described on page 19 in chapter 2, Preparing for Water Workouts: Tuck in and tighten your abdominals (the muscles that run over your entire abdomen and rib cage from your breastbone to your pelvis) and squeeze your buttocks together. Avoid tipping your pelvis under, which strains your lower back. Breathe deeply while maintaining the abdominal and buttocks tuck.

Resistance and Movement of Force

Pushing against buoyancy creates resistance that can be increased by adding larger or more buoyancy floats to the working limb. In addition, water creates balanced resistance in multiple directions because immersion in water exerts hydrostatic pressure equally on all surfaces of the body. Movement in any forward-backward or side-to-side direction meets equal resistance in both directions so that opposing muscle groups can be worked equally. A standing Side Leg Lift, for instance, works the outside of your thigh on the way out and the inside of your thigh on the way in.

The density of water creates resistance that provides the necessary physical conditioning challenge to develop increased endurance, strength, and power. When the frontal plane of your body encounters the viscosity (density) of the water, it displaces water and meets with resistance: the faster the speed is or the greater the force, the higher is the level of resistance. This property is called the *viscosity principle*. You can also employ the density of water by using flotation-based resistance equipment that requires you to push against the force created by buoyancy. The fitness principle of *progressive overload* allows you to intensify your results as you become stronger and more proficient: Gradually increase your force and speed or add resistance equipment to intensify your workout until it feels somewhat vigorous without being exhausting. (During each workout, increase only to the point where you can still maintain stable movement control and keep your torso position strong and steady. Also, avoid increasing both the number of repetitions and the resistance at the same time.) Chapter 7, Intensifying Workouts, provides specific guidelines for creating and structuring effective workouts.

Higher viscosity (or density) in the water means that the faster you move, the greater is the resistance that a moving object encounters. To harness this training principle, perform each exercise at three speeds. As in all exercise, stay within your limits; if you cannot maintain proper stability or your muscle fatigues, you have reached your limit and it's time to switch to another move or to stop and stretch. Respecting your limits, enhancing muscle balance, moving in multiple directions, and moving at multiple speeds are key principles in physical conditioning for healthy function, the optimal goal of fitness.

Key Exercise Principles for Healthy Function

Water fitness and rehabilitation expert Igor Burdenko makes the following recommendations to achieve physical conditioning for healthy function:

1. Respect your limits. Switch exercises or stop if your muscle fatigues or you can no longer keep your position properly stabilized.
2. Enhance muscle balance by moving in multiple directions. Perform each movement in several directions.
3. Move at multiple speeds. Perform each movement using three different speeds.

Hydrostatic Pressure

Fluid pressure is exerted equally on all surface areas of an immersed body at rest at a given depth. Water exerts a force even on a stationary body. This force assists blood flow back to the heart, so it lowers blood pressure and heart rate compared to the results of performing the same activity on land. This hydrostatic pressure around the joints and the spine also makes stretching more comfortable and easier to achieve because the equalized pressure can relieve the tension in the joint and allow the tissues around the joint to relax, hence allowing for greater stretching comfort and results. Hydrostatic pressure also means that your body encounters resistance in all directions, creating an opportunity for using your muscles in strength-building motions that match the true "functional" motions you use in everyday life, rather than the contrived positions and pathways of movement you are restricted to when using most fitness training equipment. As a result, you can do a much better job in water of improving what is called functional strength, the ability to use your body through a multitude of functional actions encountered day to day.

Leverage and Eddy Drag

All movable joints in the body function as levers. You can change intensity by using your levers in several ways. Generally speaking, longer levers produce greater workload. For example, by bending your knee while gliding your leg forward and back, you shorten the lever, decrease the leverage, and reduce the intensity. This is called the *leverage principle*.

You can also change your body position to increase or decrease the body's surface area to take advantage of turbulent *eddy drag* (the circular currents created when you move in water). The flow of water may be either streamlined or turbulent. Turbulence is created when you move an unstreamlined shape through the water, thus increasing resistance. Alternately, streamlined shapes produce a steady, smooth movement of the water. For example, walking with your hands on your hips creates more eddy drag and turbulence than walking with your arms at your sides.

Putting These Concepts Into Practice

Notice that, during your exercise sequence, a Can-Can Kick with a straight leg meets with more resistance than a Knee-Lift Jog or March. To reduce intensity, bend the limb that is moving in a forward or backward direction (see figure 1.2*a*). During side-to-side movements, however, bending your limbs increases resistance (see figure 1.2*b*). The bent limb intensifies the workload of Floating Side Scissors, Step Wide Side, or Side Arm Pump by increasing the turbulence encountered by the movement of the bent limb. Other ways to increase your frontal resistance include cupping your hands to catch the water or adding equipment. The more water that you scoop up (the greater the surface area) with cupped hands, webbed gloves, paddles, or resistance bells, the harder you have to work to move the watery load.

This wide array of water attributes can be woven into the poetry of movement in water to create effective and satisfying water workouts. Buoyancy lifts your body and your spirit, liberates your joints from the downward pressure of gravity, and brings bouncy fun and strengthening resistance. Smoothly pushing through the viscosity of water both calms and challenges you while it burns more calories and empowers greater strength and cardiorespiratory fitness results in less time. The equalized resistance in all directions created

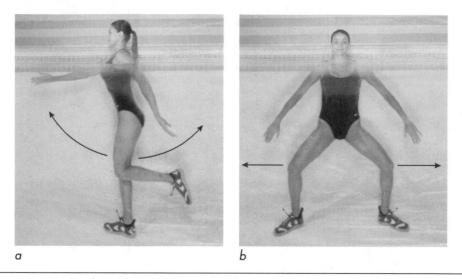

a   b

Figure 1.2 During forward and backward leg movements, reduce intensity by (a) bending your limbs. During side-to-side movements, (b) a bent limb will increase intensity by creating turbulence that elevates resistance.

by hydrostatic pressure frees your body to gain functional strength that can reduce pain, heighten performance, and improve your overall quality of life. And stirring up the water with the turbulence of eddy drag ignites excitement and challenge that spurs your body on to higher levels of fitness by charging up the intensity. Integrate these potent principles throughout each workout to capture the unique advantages of water.

CHAPTER 2

Preparing for Water Workouts

Before beginning, consider several key ways to heighten enjoyment and maximize fitness success. Learn how to reduce injury risk, ensure safety, sequence a water workout session, prepare the environment, and incorporate water exercise equipment into workouts. Review these guidelines again before beginning your first water workout to make sure you have made all of the appropriate preparations. By following these steps, you will be more satisfied with your experience and avoid circumstances that could get in the way of your continued success with water workouts.

Safety and Injury Prevention

As with any new exercise program, before you begin, check with your doctor, who can provide recommendations appropriate to your individual situation. Although most people can benefit from water exercise, readers should be aware of several situations in which it is advisable to avoid pool exercise:

- Fever
- Urinary infection
- Open wound
- Infectious disease
- Contagious skin rash
- Extreme fear of water
- Recent heart problems (Obtain medical approval and guidance.)

Fortunately, most of these conditions tend to be temporary in nature and present only a passing obstacle to beginning a water exercise program. If you are in doubt as to whether or not water exercise is right for you, consult your physician or health professional.

Adapting to a New Exercise Program

Your body needs to adapt gradually to your new water fitness program. Even if you have been exercising regularly, you are introducing your body to a different and new demand, and it must adapt and grow to meet the challenge gradually. This process of adaptation is what increases the level of fitness. Gradual introduction is especially essential for people who have been inactive (exercising fewer than two or three times a week during the past several years), injured, or ill. If that is your situation, get your doctor's approval first. Then start out with some simple water striding for 5 to 10 minutes (walking) and static stretching two or three times a week for the first few weeks. Then add 1 minute each week and allow your body to develop the basic level of fitness that is required before more strenuous exercise can be attempted without risk of overuse injury or illness. To avoid discouraging and painful setbacks, follow the Initial Conditioning Stage guidelines on the next page before trying more vigorous activity.

To prevent injury, always use stabilized posture and controlled movements, especially while exercising with equipment. Some movements require reduced speed to maintain adequate control of body position and postural alignment. To further decrease chances of impact shock injury—from striking your foot against the bottom of the pool—use flotation belts, buoys, vests, and other specially designed equipment during aerobic conditioning. When performing shallow water exercise for aerobic conditioning, begin with smaller movements and increase the size of your movements as you become more fit. Even if you are already fit, you should increase your intensity gradually, over a period of weeks or months, to avoid injuries, illness, and chronic fatigue. Overuse problems can result if you don't give your body enough time to become adequately conditioned in response to the newly introduced demands of water exercise.

Initial Conditioning Stage

To develop a basic level of fitness, begin with low-intensity water striding or walking, slowly performed range-of-motion exercise, complete body stretches, and light calisthenics. Starting out slowly and gradually minimizes muscle soreness and exercise discomfort. Monitor your heart rate to be sure you are exercising at the low end of your target heart rate zone. In terms of perceived exertion, your intensity level should feel "moderate or somewhat hard." If you have not previously been exercising at all, exercise lightly for 5 minutes three times a day. When you are ready, follow this initial conditioning program:

1. Using a pattern of exercising every other day, warm up with water walking.
2. Stretch.
3. Complete 10 to 15 minutes of moderate aerobic exercise such as water walking, followed by cool-down and stretch. Proper stretching helps minimize soreness.

If you are just starting out, you may need from 4 to 10 weeks of initial conditioning before beginning more vigorous exercise.

Injury Prevention Checklist

The most important information in this book is contained in the Injury Prevention Checklist on the following pages. If you read the guidelines carefully and reacquaint yourself with them regularly, you will have a much better exercise experience. Before long, these techniques become automatic, like the skills needed for driving a car or riding a bicycle.

Injury Prevention Checklist

- To protect the structures of your body from injury, maintain the "braced neutral position" (figure 2.1) during all exercises, stretches, and movements. The braced neutral position helps you maintain postural stability and prevents injury, particularly to the back. An estimated 80 percent of the population is vulnerable to chronic back pain. Use of this postural technique can help you avoid a debilitating and painful common health problem.

  - Stand with your feet shoulder-width apart and your legs relatively straight, but with your knees not locked.
  - Align your pelvis in the neutral position, not tilted forward or backward.
  - Perform the "rock belly": Take a deep breath. As you exhale, contract or shorten the muscles of your abdomen. The abdominus rectus

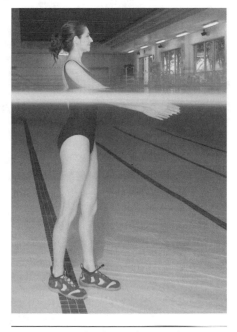

Figure 2.1 The braced neutral position helps prevent back, hip, and knee pain and represents the foundation for every exercise you will perform.

(continued)

Injury Prevention Checklist *(continued)*

muscle runs from your breastbone to your pelvis. Think of compressing the long muscles between your breastbone and your pelvis, like closing an accordion. Tighten the muscles over and under your rib cage. You will gradually develop a natural strength that allows you to keep your abdominal muscles firmly contracted automatically during exercise and movement.

- At the same time, lightly squeeze the muscles of your buttocks together in order to brace your spine in the neutral position.
- Lift and "open" your chest and keep your shoulders back and relaxed (avoid hunching your shoulders). Keep your shoulders in a straight line over your hips.
- Stand up straight, with your torso erect and your rib cage lifted.
- Keep your head level (avoid tilting your head back or forward), with your ears over your shoulders.
- Breathe deeply and evenly.
- Remind yourself frequently to return to the braced neutral position and the "rock belly" to protect your back during jumps, leaps, and stretches, toning exercises, knee lifts, and many other exercises, particularly those that require you to reach overhead or press your legs back behind you.

- Remember to breathe properly. It sounds simple, but it is very easy to forget and hold your breath while you concentrate on everything else. Oxygen is an essential ingredient in the energy fueling process. Breathe deeply and evenly at all times to prevent injury-causing fatigue.

- Avoid hyperextending your joints. Keep your knees and elbows slightly bent when you extend (straighten) fully. This "softening" of the joints protects your joints from excessive pressure that can cause tendonitis, bursitis, or other painful injuries. Use this same technique to protect your back and your neck. Avoid overarching your back or neck (hyperextension) during kick backs, jumps, and jumping jacks, and keep your abdominal and buttock muscles tightened firmly.

- Keep your balance. To maintain your balance and protect your musculoskeletal system, move your limbs to complement one another. If you kick your right leg forward in the water, bring your left arm forward. When you press one leg back, bring both arms forward. When you kick your leg out to the right side, bring your arms to the left. Move more slowly, and reestablish the braced neutral position if you are losing your balance.

- Bring your heels all the way down. When you land with your feet directly underneath you or in front of your body following a step, jump, or other movement, bring your heels all the way down to touch the pool floor. Repeatedly raising yourself on your toes without lowering your heels can cause painful injuries similar to shin splints and tight, sore calf muscles.

- Monitor your intensity. Use the perceived exertion scale (see page 11), check your breathing, or take your pulse two or three times during your aerobic phase to see if you need to modify your intensity. To lower intensity, take smaller steps, slow down, streamline your body, or reduce the height of lifts and jumps. To increase intensity, travel more and farther; take larger steps, deeper dips, or higher jumps: alternate between high and low moves; or add resistance equipment. Faster speed is not necessarily a constructive fitness objective in the water. Working beyond your controllable speed or intensity may result in injury and overuse syndromes that discourage your progress.

- Assess your breathing to monitor your intensity. If you are not breathing a bit harder than you were when you started, you have not reached your aerobic target zone. When your breathing rate increases, your "respiration rate" indicates that you have reached the lower limit of your target zone.

- Use the "Talk Test." Can you talk? If you can still speak during your aerobic exercise phase but are breathing a bit heavier than when you are at rest, you are exercising moderately. If you can comfortably speak a few breathy words, you are exercising at the upper limits of your aerobic target zone. If you cannot speak without gasping, you have passed the anaerobic threshold and have exceeded your aerobic target zone limit; then it is time to slow down.

- Keep your muscles warm during the stretch phase. During exercise, your body rids itself of excess heat through sweat evaporation and by transferring heat to the skin where it is radiated into the environment. This process occurs more quickly in water because water dissipates heat four times more quickly and efficiently than air. Gliding movements of your arms during lower-body stretches generate body heat and keep your muscles warm for more effective stretching. Once you have developed torso stability, jog or march in place while stretching your upper-body muscles. You can omit these peripheral movements if they confuse you, throw off your stability, or irritate sensitive shoulder joints.

- Avoid bouncing stretches during warm-up and cool-down. Hold the stretch position statically (without bouncing) for 10 seconds during warm-up and 20 to 30 seconds during cool-down to lengthen your muscle safely without invoking reflexive shortening, called "the stretch reflex response." The exception to this guideline is to perform warm-up movements that imitate the actions of the sport you engage in, on land

(continued)

Injury Prevention Checklist *(continued)*

or in water. You can perform the same movements of your sport in the water, in slow motion. This technique makes for a fun warm-up, prepares your body for more vigorous activity, and improves your condition for your specific sport.

- Increase your workout gradually. You can save yourself the pain and aggravation of injury (and even the heartache of "overuse flu," a chronic cold some people experience when they exercise too much or too often) if you start with a comfortable exercise schedule (for example, three times a week for 15 to 30 minutes, including warm-up and cool-down) and then increase the time gradually. Give your body a few weeks to adapt to the new level of exercise before increasing again. Increase only in small increments and vary your avenue of increase (frequency, intensity, or duration). If you increase too much or too soon, your body may force you to stop altogether. Pain is a signal to stop exercising, seek medical attention, or revise your workout.

- Protect your wrist joint. Keep your hand in a straight line with your forearm at all times. Avoid bending your wrist forward or backward during repetitive movements against resistance (figure 2.2). In addition, when pushing your hand against the pressure of the water, always press your palms *facing* the water. Your wrist and forearm are more resilient to injury in this position, and you can harness more of the water's resistive qualities. Cup your hand for even greater resistance or use webbed gloves.

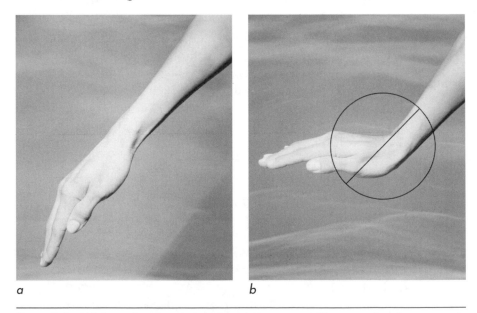

a   *b*

Figure 2.2 While pushing your hands through the water, *(a)* keep your hands in a straight line with your forearm. Avoid *(b)* bending your wrist upward.

- Strengthen your muscles through their full, pain-free, normal range of motion. Short, choppy, movements that strengthen only through a limited range of motion increase the risk of injury. Avoid overstraightening, also called hyperextension, because it indicates movement beyond the normal range of motion and ultimately leads to injury.

- Exercise your muscles evenly to produce balanced results. As described in chapter 1, Improving Fitness With Water Exercises, opposing muscle groups sustain an important relationship. Injuries result when one muscle is too strong or less flexible in relation to the opposing muscle. Therefore, work and stretch your opposing muscle groups equally to avoid injury. People often focus on the muscles in the front of the body and neglect the muscles in the back of the body. For instance, avoid overemphasizing Front Knee Lift Jog or March while overlooking Alternate Leg Press-Back, an exercise that works your lower-body muscles to the rear.

- Avoid movements that involve leaning forward without support or twisting your torso simultaneously. For example, omit exercises that require you to bring your elbows down toward your opposite raised knee. Such twisting repeatedly can put debilitating torsion stress on your spine.

Other Tips for Comfort and Safety

A comfortable bathing suit that does not bind, slip, or ride up is preferable for water exercise. Women may prefer the comfort of a bathing suit with straps that cross or connect in the back to prevent the straps from sliding. Shorts and a top (loose fitting but not too billowy) suffice if you are not using a bathing suit.

If you tend to chill easily or prefer more support than a bathing suit provides, wear a leotard and footless tights along with a sports bra and T-shirt or long-sleeved top. Aquatic specialty manufacturers such as H_2OWear (for contact information, see list on pages 37 and 38) offer another option: all-in-one water workout gear made from chlorine-resistant lycra, including tights, shorts, and bodysuits with long sleeves and full-length legs (see figure 2.3).

Aqua shoes enhance secure footing by adding tread to your step and also protect the skin on your feet. Several manufacturers offer various types of aqua shoes.

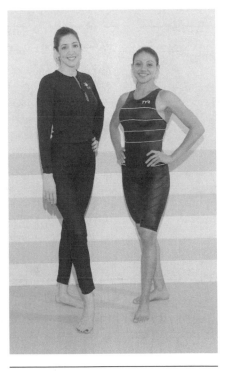

Figure 2.3 Chlorine-resistant bodysuits can help keep you warm in the water.

Shoes are essential if the pool has a rough or slippery surface or if you need more stability because of sensitive joints. People who have diabetes are more prone to foot damage and should be sure to wear aqua shoes in order to protect their feet.

Also, when exercising outdoors, protect yourself from the sun. If you exercise outdoors, wear water-resistant sunscreen to prevent sunburn, premature aging of the skin, and melanoma (skin cancer). The CDC (U.S. Centers for Disease Control) recommends SPF 15, applied 15 to 30 minutes prior to sun exposure. Pay particular attention to the back of your neck, your ears, and the areas of your scalp with thin hair. Reapply sunscreen after exiting the pool if you plan to remain outdoors. Wear 100 percent UV-ray protective sunglasses to protect your eyes from cataracts and other eye ailments. Avoid being out in the sun between 10:00 a.m. and 4:00 p.m. when the sun's rays are the most intense and likely to cause damage.

Avoid eating 1 1/2 to 2 hours prior to exercise and, when you do eat before exercise, choose easy-to-digest, low-fat foods such as whole fruit, vegetable sticks, or brown rice. Exercise shunts blood away from your stomach and digestive system and sends it instead to the working muscles. Sour stomach and food putrefaction can result.

MYTHS AND MISCONCEPTIONS

Myth: A quick sugar boost gives you more energy for your workout.

FALSE   A high-sugar snack eaten within 1 hour of exercising does not enhance your exercise energy; in fact, it has been shown scientifically to cause weakness and fatigue. Eating refined sugar triggers increased production of insulin in the blood. The insulin inhibits the metabolism of fat for energy (which makes eating sugar counterproductive if you are trying to lose fat). It also lowers the amount of sugar in the blood, which may cause you to feel a loss of energy and which may reduce the amount of exercise you can complete before fatigue stops you. In processed foods, sugar appears in many forms, such as corn syrup, dextrose, glucose, or fructose. If you seek something sweet, stick to whole fruit: Your body absorbs the natural fruit sugars gradually because of the high fiber of the whole fruit and the fact that the fruit sugar has not been refined of its natural nutrients.

To prevent chlorine from irritating your skin, shower without soap before getting into the pool. Tap water binds to your skin and helps prevent chlorine from penetrating. Then shower again after leaving the pool, this time soaping all of your skin and rinsing well. Soap helps break down the chemical bonds that link chlorine to your skin. Several manufacturers make soap and shampoo specifically designed to remove chlorine from your body: Ultra Swim, TriSwim, Soap+, WaterGear, Swimmer's Own, Swimmer's OneStep, Aubrey Organics, and Chlor-Off. Finally, use high-quality light skin lotion after every soap-and-water shower to protect your skin from loss of moisture.

The Importance of Drinking Water

Although you don't feel it as much as in land-based exercising, you do perspire during water workouts. Your body can become dehydrated during water exercise, and replenishing fluids regularly is vital for your safety.

To prevent fatigue, it is essential to keep your body hydrated before, during, and after water exercise, particularly in hot or humid environments. The best way to replace lost fluids is by drinking plain water rather than soda, juice, or coffee. These alternatives can actually contribute to dehydration because they act as diuretics, which cause the elimination of fluids. Always keep an unbreakable container filled with drinking water near the pool.

MYTHS AND MISCONCEPTIONS

Myth: You shouldn't drink water when you exercise because it gives you cramps and makes you nauseated.

FALSE   Drink eight 8-ounce (240 ml) glasses of water a day, plus two glasses one hour before and after exercising. You can drink more during exercise, especially if your activity is of long duration. Drink greater amounts of water in hot, cold, or humid weather. (Hot or humid weather makes you lose more fluids through sweat; cool weather activates the kidneys, stimulating increased urination.) Each of these conditions can cause you to become dehydrated more easily. In some cases, drinking too little can actually bring on cramping.

Environment

You will get better results and be more comfortable if you examine your exercise environment and determine how you can best suit your needs. Here are some guidelines to help prepare the best environment for your water workouts.

Temperature and Humidity

Temperature governs your comfort in water. Warm water temperatures (80 to 86 degrees Fahrenheit (27 to 30 degrees Celsius) help increase circulation to your muscles, preparing them for stretching and reducing chance of injury. (If you have arthritis, water temperatures of 83 to 86 degrees Fahrenheit [28 to 31 degrees Celsius] are preferred.) When you are not moving and creating heat as a by-product of energy production, your body may cool quickly in water, so keep your legs or arms moving to stay warm.

Temperatures above 88 degrees Fahrenheit (21 degrees Celsius) do not let your body cool down properly during aerobic activity such as water walking or Hydro Jacks: High temperatures are not recommended for a safe aerobic workout. However, nonaerobic range-of-motion exercises, such as stationary stretches, ankle or shoulder rolls, or thumb circles, performed while you are immersed in temperatures from 94 to 104 degrees Fahrenheit (34 to 40 degrees Celsius) enhance mobility and reduce the joint pain and stiffness associated with arthritis.

When you add the temperature of the water to the percentage of humidity, the end result should be below 160 to ensure your health and safety: for example, 87 degrees Fahrenheit plus 60 percent humidity equals 147. Heat-related injures and illness could result at heat and humidity sums of 160 and over. A combined temperature and humidity sum of 150 is considered the upper limit of comfortable conditions. This is a concern in both indoor and outdoor pools; you are dealing with humidity when outdoors the rest of the day and even indoor pools usually become more humid on humid days. If the day is hot and humid, reduce your intensity. If you feel lightheaded or dizzy, leave the water.

Water Depth

Perform most water workout exercises in chest-deep to waist-deep water. For more cushioning and buoyancy, seek water at chest depth. If you are overweight and deconditioned, however, you may have less control in water that is too deep; you might begin by moving more slowly or, preferably, at waist-high depths.

Deep-water flotation exercises eliminate impact entirely, providing a totally shock-free environment that allows you to increase intensity without compressing your joints. Water walking and jogging with flotation were first prescribed as rehabilitation exercise for elite athletes. Each flotation exercise pumps the cardiovascular system by using movements that use your large muscle groups (hips, buttocks, thighs) and thereby improve aerobic endurance, burn stored fat, and dissipate the negative effects of stress.

Music

Music can motivate and stimulate you to get more out of your workouts. Its smooth, continuous rhythms can help map your program from Warm-Up, through Aerobic Exercise, Muscle Strengthening and Toning, and Final Cool-Down. Often music can give you the momentum to continue on to the end of your program instead of giving up early. This music selection guide can help those who wish to exercise to music.

Select songs that have upbeat energy—songs that are full of life and make you want to move or dance. Your exercise routine is more fun if your movements interpret the music. For instance, the chorus has been described as the part "where the song blooms." You can bloom into an especially lively pattern of exercise during the chorus and then repeat the pattern each time the chorus returns. The music's energy gives you the right kind of motivation for each particular section: Invigorating energy motivates you for aerobics; a hard, steady, beat at a slow to moderate tempo drives you to continue with your strengthening moves at the right pace; and soothing energy encourages you to decrease intensity for aerobic cool-down or to soften and relax your muscles for final stretch.

Sometimes the energy stimulation that music provides is more important than whether or not you adhere to tempo. Some older adults and individuals with movement limitations need to move at the speed that is most comfortable to them at the moment. In that case, let the music entertain you rather than dictate your movement tempo. Nonrhythmic relaxation music, or recordings of bird songs, crickets, wind, rain, or waterfalls, can provide a pleasant, stimulating background for nonrhythmic movement.

Finding a Tempo

You can use the beats per minute in a piece of music to determine the tempo of your exercise. A simple way to determine the beats per minute in your favorite music is to follow these steps:

1. Find a digital watch or clock that tracks seconds, play your music, and tap your feet in time to the tempo.
2. Count the number of taps that your foot makes in 15 seconds.
3. Multiply that number by 4.

The result is the number of beats per minute in that song. Table 2.1 tells you more about matching the appropriate energy, beats per minute, and length to each section. Note that the tempo gradually increases, then decreases during the aerobic section, and finally maintains a steady beat during the calisthenics. If you are just starting out, have arthritis, are overweight, or recently have recovered from injury, be sure to use the slower tempos.

Use a tempo that gradually increases, then gradually decreases, along a bell curve, for the safest response from your heart, lungs, and circulatory system. For variation, use interval training, in which you alternate the tempo between faster and slower. Use interval training every 4 or 5 weeks: Apply the principles of interval training to boost your physical condition by challenging your cardiovascular system to work harder for a few seconds or minutes and then return to a more moderate pace for several minutes. Listen to your body: Repeat as many times as your body says you can handle it.

Safety Considerations

Avoid using plug-in appliances near the pool. Battery-operated portable musical electronics components are safer, and several manufacturers offer

Table 2.1   Set Your Routine to Music

Section	Beats per minute	# of minutes	Energy
Thermal warm-up	125-135	3-5	Stimulating
Warm-up stretch	100-135	3-5	Flowing but stimulating
Preaerobic (optional calisthenics)	115-130	3-5	Invigorating
AEROBIC EXERCISE PHASE			
Use a tempo that gradually increases, then gradually decreases, for the safest response from your heart, lungs, and circulatory system. Interval training, in which you alternate the tempo between faster and slower, is a method that highly fit exercisers can use to vary their workouts.			
Warm-up aerobic	120-135	3-5	Invigorating
Intermediate aerobic	130-145	3-5	Invigorating
Peak intensity	145-155	3-10	High energy
Intermediate aerobic	130-145	3-5	Invigorating
Cool-down aerobic	120-135	3-5	Stimulating and soothing
Calisthenics (muscle strengthening and toning exercises)	115-135	10-20	Rhythmic and stimulating
Final cool-down stretch	90-110	5-10	Soothing

rechargeable players. If you use a plug-in appliance, be sure that it is 5 or more feet (1.5 m) from the pool and elevated on a nonmetallic table or shelf and that your power cord is free from frays or exposed areas. Do not plug in, unplug, or use appliances while standing in a puddle.

If you must use a plug-in appliance near the pool, buy a ground-fault circuit interrupter (GFCI), a device designed to prevent electrocution, that can be purchased for very little cost from hardware and electrical supply stores. It comes as either a portable adapter for plugging into an outlet or as a replacement for the outlet.

Adding Equipment

With water exercise equipment, you can alter your workouts to add variety, increase intensity, or recover from injury. All equipment uses buoyancy, weight, or resistance (or a combination of these principles). Resistance and flotation tools—such as water jugs, webbed gloves, paddles, plastic plates, floats, boots, or bells—let you increase your workload as you become more fit or reduce impact to prevent or rehabilitate injuries. Various commercial devices are available, or you can recycle household items into resourceful water workout equipment. Aquatic exercise specialist Ruth Sova developed guidelines for adding equipment to workout programs for the Aquatic Exercise Association. The following guidelines build on Ruth Sova's recommendations.

Before using water exercise equipment to enhance your workout, be sure that you are thoroughly familiar with how your body moves in water. The weightlessness of exercising in water requires a new set of muscle "memories" (reflexes and automatic responses) for you to control your movements adequately and predict your body's response in the aquatic environment. Once you have adapted to the weightless environment, carefully consider which kind of equipment best suits your needs and objectives.

To prevent injury during deep-water aerobics, choose the type of flotation device that is best for you. For example, use empty gallon jugs or manufactured flotation cuffs if you do not experience neck or shoulder pain; the Wet Vest AT or upper-arm cuffs if you have not developed proficient torso muscles; a flotation belt if you have a relatively strong torso and want to include upper-body aerobic movements; foot or ankle flotation cuffs with flotation bells if you have a very strong torso and seek a nonimpact challenge; or the Wet Vest if you need maximum comfort and stability.

For muscle strength and toning, your choices in resistance equipment range from webbed gloves and water weights to handheld water resistors and lower-leg attachments. Because incorporating water exercise equipment into your workout introduces special safety concerns, you should take the following precautions for building strength and toning muscles with water exercise equipment, in addition to the guidelines provided in the "Injury Prevention Checklist" provided earlier in this chapter, to prevent injury and maximize your success:

1. Add water resistance equipment gradually, after you have established a basic level of strength without equipment and can perform the exercise, with all of your postural stabilizing muscles held in proper positioning without wavering for 12 to 15 repetitions before reaching fatigue of the muscle group. Going too far too fast may result in discomfort or even injury and may even set you back rather than quicken your progress.

2. Always warm up and stretch first, and follow every strengthening routine with flexibility cool-down stretches to avoid soreness and injuries that can result from overly tight muscles.

3. Proper body alignment is always important, but using equipment increases the chances that faulty position and technique result in injury. Use the positioning guidelines described in the "Injury Prevention Checklist" on pages 19-23.

4. The speed of your movement with resistance equipment determines the intensity level: The faster you push or pull, the heavier is the resistance. Each time you use equipment, begin slowly and add more forceful movements gradually. If you cannot maintain complete control over the movements and your body alignment, you have exceeded your maximum appropriate speed. Always use careful placement; never toss the equipment about randomly.

5. To protect your joints, use slower movements when your limbs are straight and faster movements when they are bent. Be sure to keep your elbows and knees bent slightly to avoid hyperextending (overstraightening) the joint.

6. Keep the equipment in the water. Moves that begin or end out of the water greatly increase the risk of injury to the joints.

7. Beginners should avoid exercises that require you to keep your arms or legs away from your body while you perform repetitive circles. Instead, reduce strain on the ligaments and tendons of your shoulders, knees, hips, back, and elbows by performing repetitions that bring your limbs *toward* your body instead of holding them *away* from your body.

8. Short, limited-range movements can cause injury. Choppy movements shorten muscles and only build strength in limited ranges of motion. Concentrate on using the full range of motion around a joint while maintaining proper body alignment, thus building strength throughout the entire range.

9. Never exercise in the pool by yourself. Drowning accidents are unpredictable. Avoid the risk by making sure someone is with you at the pool at all times.

Making Equipment From Household Items

Many common household items make excellent and inexpensive water workout equipment. The following examples can be fashioned inexpensively from common household items.

- **Kids' kickboards.** Use kids' kickboards to work the upper body in push and pull exercises. Small kickboards offer increased surface area and buoyancy over plates, so start without equipment and then later add the plates; graduate to kickboards when you need more resistance. Sit on a kickboard to "water taxi" around the pool while kicking your legs and pressing the water back with your arms. Sit upright, with your abdominal muscles tight and your shoulders down.

- **Old lightweight canvas sneakers.** Wear your clean old lightweight canvas sneakers in place of aquatic shoes for traction and stability. Toss them in the washing machine to remove all dirt.

- **Plastic jugs.** Empty plastic gallon jugs provide flotation for deep-water exercise and can be used to increase resistance in abdominal exercises. Hug the jugs under your arms to provide an inexpensive form of flotation. (People with neck concerns should not use jugs for flotation.) For abdominal work, hug the jugs to your chest as you stand in chest-deep water in a shoulder-width and stable stance; contract your abdominals to shorten the distance slightly between your rib cage and pelvis. The buoyancy of the jugs resists your movement and provides you with a greater challenge to strengthen your abdominal muscles. Be sure to soak off the labels on jugs to protect the pool filter. If you use milk jugs, wash them with hot, soapy water, let them dry with the caps off, and then resecure the caps.

- **Plastic picnic plates or frisbees.** Wash your family's plastic picnic plates and use them for added resistance during upper-body exercises. Frisbees also work well. Be sure to start with the smaller sizes first; you can graduate to the larger sizes as your strength develops. The two disks must be identical in size and density to ensure balanced muscle conditioning and prevent injury. To make this work, keep the water pressure constantly against the plates as you push them through the water, turning your wrists carefully and slowly to keep the pressure on as you change the direction you are pushing the plates. If you stop, the plates drop. It's easier if you push both plates in the same direction. Give yourself a break and have fun with this, because they *will* drop at first!

Commonly Used Equipment

This list focuses on the best design options available in this broad field. Use this guide to learn more about how to choose from the most frequently used commercial water exercise equipment and to get information about major aquatic equipment designs that have been introduced. The recommendations of each type of equipment and suggestions for where to obtain equipment are referenced to the numbered list of distributors and manufacturers on pages 37 and 38.

- **Aqua shoes.** Look for shoes that fit comfortably without squeezing, binding, or crushing into the top of your foot. Be sure that they fit snugly enough so that they do not slip off when you jump up in the water. Lightweight shoes with good traction add a bit of resistance and a lot of stability. Some shoes are made of wetsuit material that helps keep your feet and ankles warm. AQx Sports makes an aqua shoe with a series of small cups along the sides to scoop water and increase resistance as you press your foot back. Contact distributor 2, 7, 8, 13, 14, 16, 17 or any of several fitness shoe companies.
- **Chlorine-resistant lycra and body-warming apparel.** If you tend to chill easily, use a full bodysuit with long sleeves and long legs, which are available from distributors and manufacturers 1, 7, 10, 12, 13, 14, and 16. These vendors provide sizes and styles for men and women and also offer chlorine-resistant tights, shorts, tops, swimsuits with long or short tights attached, swim skirts with briefs, and long-sleeved neoprene jackets and tights. For warmth before and after water exercise, cover up with an aqua parka from distributor 13.
- **Flotation vests, belts, and upper arm cuffs.** Flotation devices for deep-water exercise vary from simple belts and arm or foot floats to convertible

cuffs and exercise vests. Two of the best for comfort, price, and function are the HYDRO-FIT Wave Belt (distributor 8) and the Water Gym Flotation Belt (distributors 7 and 17). The HYDRO-FIT Wave Belt forms to the natural shape of your body and has a unique contour that balances buoyancy evenly around your torso, enhancing correct posture and body alignment and reducing the feeling of being tippy or wobbly. The Wet Vest (see figure 2.4), a more expensive product, provides a very durable and comfortable option that requires less torso strength for successful vertical balance. The Wet Vest AT, a less expensive version, fits around your hips, not your waist. Built-in pants hold the

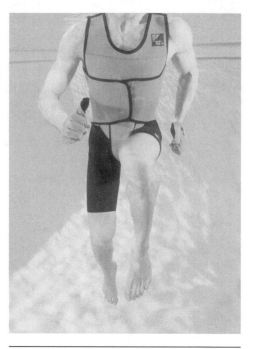

Figure 2.4 HYDRO-FIT Wet Vest.

HYDRO-FIT images provided by RIC-FRAZIER Productions.

AT comfortably in place, preventing it from riding up. The pant design includes soft, contoured edges that put little or no pressure on your ribs and allow for ease of movement. The Free Floaters product, a low-cost alternative worn on the upper arms, also requires less torso strength and works well for abdominal exercise. Sprint supplies inexpensive flotation belts and adult-sized water wings worn on the upper arms. AQx makes a flotation suit that looks like a sleeveless wetsuit, but actually makes you float. Contact distributor 2, 5, 6, 7, 8, 9, 10, 11, 12, 13, 14, 15, 16, 17, or 19.

- **Flotation noodles.** Water noodles are cheap and available everywhere. These flexible 3- to 5-foot (.9 to 1.5 m) foam noodles provide a versatile and inexpensive flotation option (see figure 2.5). Add noodle handles to enable better grip and to allow use of the noodle for muscle resistance exercise as well as flotation aerobic conditioning. Contact your local sporting goods or discount store or distributor 6, 8, 10, 13, 14, or 19.

- **Buoyant barbells, cuffs, and balls.** Barbells make a good flotation option if you do not experience hand, shoulder, neck, or upper-back pain. Use them to buoy yourself for lower-body exercise, deep-water aerobics, or abdominal exercise, or press them through the water in shallow depths to increase upper-body resistance and improve muscle fitness. Ankle cuffs fit comfortably over the ankles and provide added resistance to the lower body; some models can be used for advanced deep-water exercise in combination with flotation barbells. Swim and therapy bars, a 30-inch (76.2 cm) version of the hand bars with double floats at each end, provide stable and secure buoyancy for added support. Flotation balls add resistance to your workout and come in many sizes. Balls are especially effective for adding buoyancy resistance to abdominal crunches. HYDRO-FIT offers convertible upper-arm cuffs that can be easily fashioned into a flotation belt or ankle cuffs. Figure 2.6 illustrates buoyant barbells and ankle cuffs. Contact distributor 1, 2, 5, 6, 7, 8, 10, 11, 12, 13, 14, 15, 16, 17, or 19.

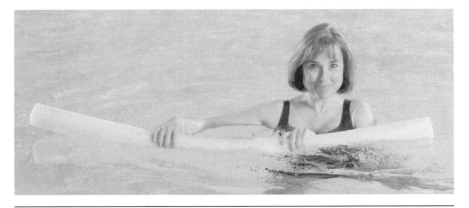

Figure 2.5 Water noodles are a versatile and inexpensive flotation option.
HYDRO-FIT images provided by RIC-FRAZIER Productions.

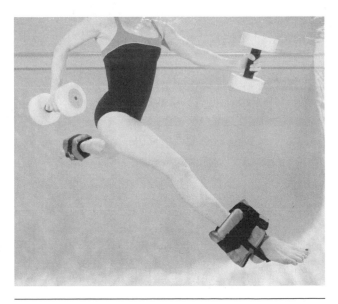

Figure 2.6 Barbells and ankle cuffs.
HYDRO-FIT images provided by RIC-FRAZIER Productions.

- **Resistance fins and flow bells.** Hydro-Tone offers a proven system that greatly magnifies the resistance of movement through water. The equipment enhances exercise for all major muscles of the body, including the heart. The degree of resistance automatically changes with the amount of effort or force you apply. To purchase this highly effective mode of water exercise, contact distributors 10, 11, or 14. For fin boots with lighter and smaller resistance at a lower cost, consider Aquafins or Mini Fins. Contact distributor 1, 9,10, 11, 14, 15, 16, or 19.

- **Webbed gloves.** Water gloves create a webbed hand to increase the water's resistance to your upper-body movements. Use webbed gloves to enhance upper-body muscle endurance and strength and to intensify your aerobic workout. Contact distributor 6, 7, 8, 9, 10, 11, 12, 13, 14, 16, 17, 18, or 19.

- **Aquatic step.** Aquatic bench stepping combines the intensity and versatility of stair climbing with the protection of an aquatic environment. The waterproof, sinkable platforms come in several heights and provide an alternative to stair-climbing machines or land-based step aerobics. The platform can also be used to alter depths in single-depth pools so that shorter people can perform Supported Squats or the Deep Muscle Hip, Thigh, and Buttocks Stretch. Speedo AquaStep makes a waterproof aerobic step platform that is lightweight yet sinks to the pool floor and offers height adjustments. Contact distributor 3, 6, 11, 12, 13, or 14.

- **Boards.** Sprint, Zura, and Burdenko make buoyant underwater boards on which you sit, kneel, or stand for dynamic movements. The boards are uniquely shaped to challenge and strengthen stability and balance in the water. One Burdenko Board version has straps and is used in both shallow and deep water to develop upper- and lower-body fitness in each essential area: balance, coordination, flexibility, endurance, speed, and strength. In addition, many distributors offer a variety of kickboards, which represent an inexpensive and versatile option for resistance, balance, and cardiorespiratory training. Contact distributor 5, 6, 11, 12, 13, 14, 15, 16, or 19.

- **Fitness vest.** The weighted X Vest helps you strengthen core muscles, improve spinal bone density, lose extra pounds safely and effectively, and maintain healthy weight. The engineering of the X Vest allows you to train your body in proper body alignment and balance. Wear the vest during water workouts to enhance results with core strengthening, aerobic moves in the shallow end of the pool, water yoga, and advanced power and plyometrics training. By using a fitness vest such as the X2, for example, you give your body a heightened challenge. Your body is currently acclimated to your weight. It burns calories based on weight, exercise, duration, and intensity. When you add weight to your body, more muscles are recruited to support the function of moving; in turn, more calories are burned to support the muscle action, increasing your metabolic rate so that you burn more calories in the same amount of time, making your workout more effective. Contact distributor 18.

- **Burdenko exercise belt.** The Burdenko Belt is an all-in-one resistance invention designed for use on land or in the water. Use this amphibious tool for a complete body workout that can provide aerobic conditioning, balance, coordination, flexibility, and strength. Surgical tubing extends from the belt to work your arms, legs, and torso. The belt is simple to adjust and serves as a back support. This highly versatile workout belt is ideal for use in a home gym and convenient for travel. Contact distributor 5.

- **Water walkers.** By wearing flexible foot paddles called winged water walkers, you can burn two to three times as many calories per minute as you do in standard water jogging or jogging on land. (Walking with water walkers burns 20 to 22 calories per minute compared to 11 calories per minute for standard water jogging or 8 calories per minute for land jogging.) Flexible paddles strap to the feet. Wings on the sides of the paddles unfold to form a wider surface for increased resistance during the downward movement and then refold for minimal resistance during upward movement. Wear water walkers with a flotation belt or vest and use them to strengthen core muscle groups, the abdominals, gluteals (buttocks), and hip flexors. Winged water walkers provide a challenging physical conditioning method for athletes and an efficient workout for people who are recovering from surgery or injury, are overweight or obese, are older adults, or have chronic conditions such as arthritis, asthma, and fibromyalgia. Contact distributor 5, 14, or 17.

- **Water weights.** Waterproof weights come in varying degrees of heaviness or can be adjustable. Some attach to your wrists or ankles; others are handheld. Use them to enhance upper-body toning. Wear a flotation vest or belt and attach the weights to your ankles to provide lower-body resistance or to hang suspended without motion in order to release pressure on your lower back, open up your spinal joints, and lengthen your spine. Weights are not recommended for use during aerobic exercise or other quick movements. Contact distributor 1, 7, 9, 10, 11,12, 13, or 14.

- **Cast guards and limb splints.** Cast guards keep casts and bandages dry while submersed in water. They are available in shapes to fit arms, legs, hands, and feet and in sizes for men, women, and children. Latex construction provides a strong, durable, and tear-resistant fit over wounds, sores, and all types of casts. Limb splints keep joints still so that the resistance of the water does not bend sore or injured joints (e.g., elbow or knee) that need to remain immobile while the muscles of a nearby joint (e.g., shoulder or hip) move the limb through the water. Contact distributor 5 for cast guards and distributor 14 for aqua limb splints.

- **AquaTunes.** This water sport belt holds your personal cassette, CD, or MP3 player so that you can keep moving to the music when in the water.

To use it, insert the mini-electronics in the waterproof pouch, close the watertight seal, and perform your workout. AquaTunes comes with an earplug speaker system that secures the speaker in your ear and keeps water out of your ear. The clear PVC enables better visibility and operation of controls. For the AquaTunes water sport belt, contact distributor 17.

Specialized Equipment

The popularity of water exercise has brought new inventions to the marketplace. Several distributors have developed specialized strength stations and cardiorespiratory or aerobic training machines that take advantage of the properties of the aquatic environment. Devices that can enhance your water workout have become available as well, including hardware to assist in balance for water walking.

- **Water workout stations.** The Aquatrend water workout station is a resistance training station for your pool that uses the mass of your body and the density of the water to improve functional strength in a way that is not possible on land (figure 2.7). Ordinary land-based fitness machines require that you make adjustments to the machine in order to match your body characteristics; the adjustment capabilities of many of the machines can only provide a good fit for a small segment of people who fall into a certain range of size and joint geometry. The design of the Aquatrend station allows the user to strengthen, tone, and improve joint mobility in ways that match each person's natural functional movements, regardless of his or her size or shape. The station can be used successfully at home or in rehabilitation, conditioning, and training programs. The Aquatrend workout programs reach more than 600 muscles in the human body; they free users from the limitations of gravity. For chin-ups, for example, this equipment buoys your body weight just enough to assist the movement so that you can perform it with proper technique, in comfort, and without strain. A wide variety of uses include stretching muscles, working on pelvic stability, and achieving body alignment. Contact distributor 1, 4, or 6.

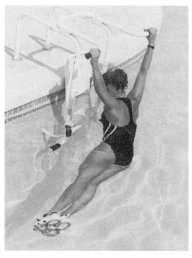

Figure 2.7 The Aquatrend resistance training station expands functional, strength, and flexibility training options in the pool.

Photo courtesy of Aqua Trends.

- **Aqua bike.** Submersible aquatic stationary cycles make it possible to pedal against the smooth, natural resistance of water. Settings for five levels of workout intensity allow the user to upgrade training programs or to personalize for beginner, intermediate, and advanced levels. When choosing an aquatic bike, make sure that it has an adjustable saddle seat and handlebars so that it can be set up to match each user's personal body geometry and therefore prevent injury caused by inappropriate seating position. For aquatic cycles, contact distributor 3, 6, 14, or 15.

- **Aqua treadmill.** There are many aquatic treadmill options. Aquatic Therapy Source (ATS) treadmills use a flat, nonmotorized walking deck and a nearly frictionless walking belt. The user determines the speed by walking or running at the desired pace; the walking belt reacts in a match to the input it receives from the user's feet. Resistance is produced by the surface area of the user's body moving through the water and dramatically increases with the slightest increase in the striding rate. This particular treadmill does not have electromechanical or electronic components that can fail quickly in the pool environment, rollers that can cause injury to the soles of the feet, or treadmill belt tracking adjustments or mechanism (the belt system is self-tracking). There is a walking deck close to the pool floor that allows for chest-height submersion in pools that are only 4 feet (1.2 m) deep. For underwater treadmills, contact distributor 1, 3, 11, 14, or 15.

- **Water walking assistant.** Sprint's water walking assistant represents a low-cost instrument that can improve your balance and gait by increasing leg and torso strength. The relatively inexpensive flotation frame provides support to your arms and upper body and has padded handles for a comfortable grip. For the water walking assistant, contact distributor 14.

Equipment Distributors and Manufacturers

1. ActiveForever — Web site: www.activeforever.com/Products
Toll free: 800-377-8033

2. AQX Sports — Web site: www.aqxsports.com
Toll free: 800-203-1276

3. Aquatic Therapy Source — Web site: www.pooltherapy.com
(Phone number is not available.)

4. Aquatic Trends Inc. — Web site: www.aquatictrends.com
Toll Free: 800-775-9588

5. Burdenko Water and Sports Therapy Institute — Web site: www.burdenko.com
Phone: 781-862-3727

6. Excel Sports Science — Web site: www.aquajogger.com
Toll Free: 800-922-9544

7. H_2O Wear — Web site: www.h2owear.com
Toll free: 800-321-7848

  8. HYDRO-FIT
     Web site: www.hydrofit.com
     Toll free: 800-346-7295

  9. Hydro-Tone International
     Web site: www.hydro-tone.com/
     products.html
     Toll free: 800-622-8663

10. Jun Konno -
    Aqua Dynamics Institute
     Web site: www.aqua-adi.co.jp
     Phone: +81-45-544-9098 (Japan)

11. Recreonics
     Web site: www.recreonics.com
     Toll free: 800-428-3254

12. Speedo
     Web site: www.speedousa.com
     Toll free: 888-477-3336

13. Splash International
     Web site: www.splashinternational.com
     Toll free: 888-775-2744

14. Sprint-Rothhammer
    International
     Web site: www.sprintaquatics.com
     Toll free: 800-235-2156

15. Thera-Band
     Web site: www.thera-band.com
     Toll free: 800-321-2135 (U.S.A. only)
     Phone: 330-633-8460
     (outside the U.S.A.)

16. Tyr Sport Inc.
     Web site: www.tyr.com
     Phone: 714-897-0799

17. WaterWorkOut
     Web site: www.waterworkout.com
     Toll free: 800-566-2182

18. The X Vest
     Web site: www.thexvest.com
     Toll free: 800-697-5658

19. Zura Sports
     Web site: www.zura.com
     Toll free: 800-890-3009

CHAPTER 3

Understanding the Phases of a Water Workout

It's a good idea to build an understanding of the basic principles that affect your body's ability to become more fit and enhance functional capacity. Fitness principles provide the fundamental tools for enhancing your level of fitness. Use these tools to make sound workout choices and effective fitness plans, whether you are introducing fitness into your lifestyle or adding water workouts into your existing fitness program.

Fitness Principles

Tissues adapt to the load to which they are exposed. Therefore, to become more fit and increase functional capacity, use the *overload principle*. The muscles, including the heart, get stronger if you gradually place greater demands on them than they are used to performing. The concept of overload originates in ancient Greek mythology with the story of Milo of Crotona, who wished to become the strongest man in Greece. As a youth, he began lifting a young bull every day; as the bull grew, so did Milo's strength. He eventually developed enough strength to lift the bull when it was full grown. This method is referred to as *progressive resistance exercise*.

The overload principle refers to this dynamic characteristic of living creatures: If a tissue or organ system is challenged to work against a load greater than usual, it becomes more fit and capable (as long as the challenge is not excessive enough to cause injury and the technique is safe and appropriate). For instance, if you stretch a muscle a little longer or more often than it is used to being stretched, it becomes more flexible. If you exercise a bit longer or more intensely than you are accustomed to exercising, your muscular or cardiorespiratory endurance increases. More repetition or greater resistance challenges the muscles and they become stronger and more firm. Injury occurs if you take the overload principle too far.

The variables that contribute to overload include frequency, intensity, type, and time (duration) of the exercise, sometimes referred to as the *FITT principle*. The key for success is to increase in only one dimension (frequency, intensity, or duration) at a time and by only a small margin, 5 to 10 percent of the previous level. If you are trying out a new type of exercise, start out with lower intensity, shorter time, and perhaps less frequency than you would with a form of exercise that you have been engaging in regularly for some time. People often become injured when they increase by too much, too soon, or in too many dimensions at once.

The *reversibility principle* says that your fitness level gradually declines if you become inactive. If you do not exercise a system, muscle, or organ sufficiently and regularly, you can lose your fitness adaptations: In other words, use it or lose it. If you skip a few days or weeks of your workout, don't worry—you can eventually return to your original program, but it is important to start back gradually. Jumping right back into your program at the level you exercised before you took a break can, and often does, produce injuries.

Exercise specificity means that you must perform an exercise activity that specifically works the fitness component, body system, and muscles that you want to enhance. For example, you must perform aerobic exercise activity to strengthen the aerobic energy system, burn fat, or increase the endurance of the cardiovascular system; you perform hamstring flexibility exercises to increase the flexibility of your hamstrings. When you overload the abdominal muscles to increase their strength, you do not produce any benefit to your cardiovascular system in the form of increased aerobic fitness. The reason is that the type of training determines the effect and the muscles being used. The muscles used to run become more resistant to fatigue by running, not by strength training.

Workout Structure

The water workout is designed to enhance physical fitness, elevate physical capacity, and improve your overall health and quality of life. To realize the potential gains from your workout—including cardiorespiratory endurance, body composition, flexibility, muscular endurance, and muscular strength—you should construct your program according to a physiologically determined format. This format gradually introduces the musculoskeletal and cardiovascular systems to greater challenge, thus reducing the risk of soreness, injury, or illness.

1. **Thermal Warm-Up.** Each time you exercise, begin with a warm-up routine of movements with low to moderate speed and range of motion. The movements help you tune into your body and increase blood flow to your muscles.

2. **Warm-Up Stretch.** Warm muscles stretch easier. Follow the Thermal Warm-Up with the stretch sequence to prepare your muscles for more intense exercise and to prevent injury.

3. **Aerobic Exercise.** Aerobic exercise improves cardiorespiratory endurance and body composition. The aerobics component consists of continuously performed large movements that keep your heart rate elevated into the aerobic target zone. Start with an aerobic warm-up of mild intensity to let your body adapt to the demand of the cardiorespiratory exertion and to prevent an adverse response to the shock of sudden high-intensity activity. Gradual cool-down activity at the end of aerobic exercise is essential because it gradually reduces your heart rate and prevents excessive pooling of blood in your arms and legs.

4. **Muscle Strengthening and Toning.** If you position the aerobic section of your workout before muscle strengthening and toning, your stabilizer muscles will be ready and able to do their job properly during aerobics rather than being already tired, because strengthening exercises take your muscle to the point of fatigue. These exercises increase muscular strength and endurance in specific muscle groups, increase lean muscle tissue mass, improve body composition, and raise your rate of metabolism.

5. **Final Cool-Down Stretch.** The water workout sequence ends with a final cool-down consisting of stretching and relaxation exercises to reduce your heart rate further, prevent muscle soreness, increase flexibility, and reestablish your body's equilibrium.

MYTHS AND MISCONCEPTIONS

Myth: It was thought to be dangerous for people with high blood pressure to participate in strength training.

FALSE Studies have clearly demonstrated that strength training does not increase high blood pressure and can actually reduce blood pressure levels over time as tissues become leaner and metabolism improves. However, be sure to *breathe* when performing resistance training. Holding your breath causes the *Valsalva maneuver*, which raises blood pressure and can be dangerous or even fatal. Therefore, inhale and exhale deeply and smoothly during your entire workout, especially during the strengthening and toning sequence. When elevated blood pressure may be a concern, use lower resistance, slow the pace, and increase the number of repetitions to reduce strain and avoid potentially higher blood pressure. Always check with a doctor before beginning any workout routine, particularly if you have a personal or family history of high blood pressure.

Appropriate technique, body alignment, joint protection, proper warm-up, cool-down, stretch, and gradual progression each contribute significantly to producing injury-free, productive fitness results. The sections that follow explain how to incorporate each of these factors into a full water workout. The Basic Water Workout is a 45- to 60-minute workout designed to exercise every part of your body. It follows the prescribed sequence outlined in table 3.1.

Table 3.1   Basic Water Workout

Exercise component	Duration
Thermal warm-up	3-5 minutes
Warm-up stretch to prevent injury	3-5 minutes
Aerobic exercise—Warm-up, moderate level, peak intensity, moderate, and cool-down	15-30 minutes
Muscle strengthening and toning	5-15 minutes
Final cool-down stretches	5-10 minutes

Thermal Warm-Up

Your program begins with a thermal, rhythmic warm-up to prepare your body for exercise. During the Thermal Warm-Up, your muscles increase somewhat in temperature and become more elastic as a result of increased blood flow to the working muscles. Your joints gradually become more lubricated, to allow for comfort through a greater range of motion. The warm-up helps prepare your body for the challenge of greater intensity and makes your muscles more pliable for static stretching. Preexercise warm-up generally begins with low to moderate speed movements in the pool to raise your body temperature. You can find many warm-up moves, with illustrations of the movements, in chapter 5, Benefiting From Aerobic Moves, (see moves 1-11 and 31-35). The Thermal Warm-Up elevates your body's energy production rate, increases blood flow and oxygen to the working muscles, and improves the responsiveness of your muscles prior to stretching.

The warm-up also enhances the reactions by your nervous system, cardio-pulmonary system (heart, lungs, and circulatory system), and tendons and ligaments. These effects reduce your risk of injury because they improve coordination, delay fatigue, and make your body tissues less susceptible to damage.

Warm-Up Stretch

Stretching warmed muscles feels better than stretching muscles that are cold, and stretching reduces the risk of injury. Hold a steady, static, nonbouncing stretch, and lengthen the muscles only to the point of comfortable resistance. However, more is not better; pain is a signal that the stretch is too severe. Loosen up the stretch or review the exercise description and illustration and examine your position to see if it needs to be adjusted. See chapter 4, Warming Up and Cooling Down for the entire sequence of warm-up stretches. Perform every stretch during each workout to ensure overall flexibility.

Limit your warm-up stretches to 10 seconds each to avoid overstretching. Injuries may result if you stretch beyond your normal range of motion, bounce a stretch, or use a position that puts undue stress on your back or joints. If you are conditioned for sports, you can prepare your body by rehearsing the sport's movements after stretching statically and before reaching aerobic intensity. During cool-down stretching, work on flexibility by holding stretches longer, about 20 seconds each. Stretch to the comfortable point of resistance, breathe deeply, and follow position instructions carefully.

Aerobic Exercise

The purpose of the aerobics segment is to improve your cardiorespiratory endurance and to train your body to burn fat by challenging the heart, the lungs, and the delivery system that sends oxygen to your working muscles. To achieve this goal, work toward maintaining your heart rate continuously or discontinuously at a moderate aerobic intensity for a total of 30 minutes five days per week, with a minimum of 10 minutes per bout. Or, do rigorous aerobic activity for 20 minutes a day, three days per week. Movements that engage the larger muscle groups of the body and that you can maintain rhythmically over time produce aerobic conditioning. Swimming, cross-country skiing, walking, hiking, running, and bicycling all qualify as aerobic exercise.

Your body tells you how hard to work. Use the self-monitoring methods described in Cardiorespiratory and Aerobic Endurance on pages 7-12 in chapter 1, Improving Fitness With Water Exercises, to be sure that you are working at an appropriate rate of aerobic intensity. Exercise at an overall moderate rate if you want to lose weight or get back in shape. Pursue moderate levels of aerobic exercise to avoid triggering the fatigue that results from engaging your anaerobic sugar-burning system and to prevent injury from stress and overuse. Moderate exercise has earned enthusiasm and support from the exercise and medical communities. High-intensity aerobic activity was shown to be associated with somewhat greater cardiovascular benefits, but also with an increase in exercise-related injuries. Extensive studies have shown that moderate levels of aerobic exercise clearly produce excellent results for enhancement of longevity and prevention of illness.

Vary Intensity

Vary the intensity of your aerobics to challenge your body systems gradually and to allow them to cool down gradually. Start with an aerobic warm-up, using the warm-up moves in chapter 4, Warming Up and Cooling Down, and chapter 5, Benefiting From Aerobic Moves. Progress slowly into intermediate movements, then increase gradually to peak intensity, followed by an eased descent into intermediate aerobics, and finish with an aerobic cool-down.

This sequence—building intensity gradually, followed by a gradual lessening of intensity—is very important for protecting your cardiovascular system from abrupt changes that could trigger an adverse cardiovascular event and to prevent soreness and injury. Abruptly ceasing vigorous aerobic exertion can cause pooling of blood in the limbs, which puts unnecessary strain on your heart while your body works to divert the blood back to your trunk. Bringing your aerobic activity to a halt while you are still in peak intensity also stops your body from using up a by-product of intense aerobic activity, *lactic acid*, which lodges in your muscles and makes you feel sore the next day if you don't use it up by taking time to lower the intensity gradually over several minutes or more. Raise intensity by gradually speeding up the pace of movements, using eddy drag (push larger surface through water) or leverage (longer levers produce more resistance). Table 3.2 provides a recommended aerobic progression.

Change Movements Gradually

Change gradually from one movement to the next to give your body a chance to adjust safely. Smooth transitions cut your risk of injury. Gliding easily from movement to movement takes practice, but it's worth the effort and

Table 3.2   Suggested Aerobic Progression

Aerobic warm-up and intermediate aerobics	Start out with easy continuous movements that work the larger muscles. This gradual increase of activity allows the cardiovascular and musculoskeletal systems to adjust gradually to increasing exercise demands. Keep movements smaller and slower in the beginning; then gradually quicken the pace, use larger movements, and cover more territory while moving about the pool.
Peak aerobics	Now that you have gradually built your intensity, continue exercising at this elevated heart rate. Use large, controlled movements, change direction, travel around the pool, vary high and low steps, use jumps and flutter kicks, and maintain a high intensity within your working range.
Intermediate aerobics and aerobic cool-down	Many people forget to cool down gradually by progressively changing to smaller movements, reducing travel about the pool, and lessening impact by eliminating jumping motions. The aerobic cool-down allows the body to readjust gradually to lower intensity, lessening the risk of damage to the cardiovascular system. Cardiac complications occur most often when exercise ceases abruptly, so continue to lower your heart rate gradually to 120 beats per minute or the low end of your target zone, whichever is lower. Gradual cool-down helps prevent excessive pooling of blood in the extremities, prevents dizziness, and reduces muscle soreness. Avoid calf soreness by bringing your heels all the way down to the floor on each landing whenever your body position allows. Drinking enough water also helps prevent muscle cramping.

comes naturally after a short time. You can make transitions more easily if you use a simple move between two complex actions. In other words, alternate between simple exercises (Pedal Jog, Hydro Jacks, Knee Lift Jog or March, Kick Up Your Heels) and more complex movements (Step Wide Side, Rocking Horse, Cross-Country Ski). See chapter 5, Benefiting From Aerobic Moves, and chapter 7, Intensifying Workouts, for exercise instructions and photographs.

Some transitions are called *progressions* because you add to the exercise by changing only one aspect of your movement at a time. For example, begin a movement of your arms without changing the movement of the legs and then change the direction or height of the exercise.

The key is to avoid changing too many aspects at once. Adding changes one by one is more comfortable and enables you to exercise smoothly and continuously. The various types of changes made during transitions include the following:

- Upper-body action changes
- Lower-body action changes
- Stationary activity versus traveling moves from place to place
- Directional changes (turn or travel left, right, front, back)
- Forward or backward moves versus lateral moves (side to side)
- Changes in movement height (high, low, medium)
- Vertical versus horizontal flotation

You can pyramid your changes by building a simple action step-by-step into a more complex movement. Add new transitions one-by-one to your original, simple move to build a pyramid. Or continuously change various aspects of your movements to progress through a variety of motions. Variety keeps you motivated, works your muscles in balance, and prevents you from overworking one muscle group while neglecting another.

Exercise Precautions

Balance the amount of exercise of the various muscle groups by using movements to the front, back, and sides and on various diagonals. Exercisers often forget to work the muscles on the sides and back of the body. Remind yourself often to press back, kick side, and kick up your heels (Back Leg Curl). Figure 3.1 illustrates examples of front, side, and back movements for overall conditioning balance. Vary stresses on the joints by alternating movements frequently, such as every 8 or 16 counts. The objective during the aerobic section is to choose exercises that challenge different muscle groups rather than reusing the same muscle group repeatedly in the same way. Focus on maintaining the braced neutral position during all aerobic exercise, particularly when you are jumping, landing, or raising your arms.

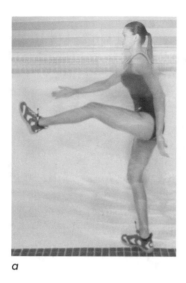

a

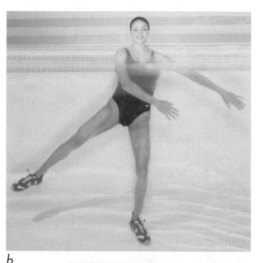

b

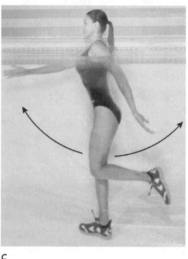

c

Figure 3.1 Balance your workout by working (a) your front muscles, (b) your side muscles, and (c) your rear muscles.

Muscle Strengthening and Toning

Toning serves as the major objective for many exercisers. However, balanced muscle strengthening can also enhance resilience to injury, increase muscle endurance, and aid in weight control by improving your lean-to-fat tissue ratio. (Fat cannot become muscle, nor can muscle become fat. Fat must be burned aerobically, and muscle tissue is developed by performing strengthening and endurance exercise.)

If you need to protect a previously injured or sensitive area, perform more repetitions at lower resistance to encourage pain-free benefits. To build maximum strength, use higher resistance and fewer repetitions. Add resistance by employing your own body weight or by using resistance equipment. Coordinate flexibility training, gradual progression, and appropriate warm-up with strength training to ensure adequate injury prevention.

MYTHS AND MISCONCEPTIONS

Myth: Women should avoid strength training because it will result in big bulky muscles.

FALSE   Because of differences in hormone levels between men and women, only men develop large bulky muscles. Women must take male hormones (steroids) in order to build large muscles; however, illicit steroid use is illegal for both women and men because of the many severe dangers of abusing anabolic steroids.

Core strength is the term used to describe the aspect of fitness that you develop by improving the stabilizing functions of your pelvic girdle (the muscles, tendons, and ligaments of your abdomen, back, buttocks, hips, and thighs) and the joints of your entire musculoskeletal system. Core strength is particularly important for preventing and overcoming injuries and helps maintain your ability to function well in daily life, even into the elder years. Improved core strength also enhances sports performance and prevents falls. Each of the strengthening segments described here contains important stabilization tips for improving core strength.

Abdominals

Abdominal and torso exercise represents one of the most universally beneficial fitness activities you can pursue. Although abdominal exercise can't give you a trimmer waistline (only regular aerobic exercise and an energy-balanced, nutritious diet that is high in vegetables and fruits and low in fat can do that), it is essential for good posture, prevention of lower-back injury, and adequate support for the stomach and intestines. The abdominal muscle group (figure 3.2) flexes, rotates, and contracts your trunk. Your body uses the abdominal muscle group all day long to protect your pelvic and spinal joints as you perform daily tasks, hence its central role in core strength. Strong abdominals contribute to the stability of your trunk and pelvis, which is crucial to long-term injury prevention, physical mobility, and independence in later life.

Water is the ideal environment for abdominal exercise because it can protect your back from injury during the challenges of gaining sleek and strong abdominal muscles. In the water, buoyancy allows defiance of gravity, a main culprit in the onset of back pain. Long periods spent in a sitting position and the downward pressure of gravity create the most common mechanisms for the origin of back pain. Buoyancy takes stress off the joints involved in almost any movement performed in the water; in the case of abdominal exercises, buoyancy takes the stress off the spinal joints.

Many people find land-based abdominal exercises difficult and ineffective. Control is awkward for beginners, and even some experienced exercisers expose themselves to injury by jerking their necks forward or arching their backs while straining to achieve results. Water workout abdominal exercises

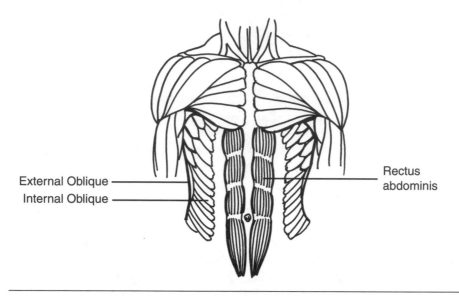

External Oblique

Internal Oblique

Rectus
abdominis

Figure 3.2 The muscles of the abdomen include the rectus abdominis and the external and internal obliques.

enable you to use water's resistance in the protective environment of aquatic buoyancy. With the appropriate techniques, you can build strength by working your abdominal muscles both alone or in coordination with your back and hips. Learn about muscle control, positioning, and breathing by performing the abdominal exercises described in chapter 6, Strengthening and Toning.

Exercise Precautions   Avoid exercises that force your back into unprotected hyperextension (lower-back arch) during movement. Unless you are at an advanced level of fitness, avoid exercises that require holding water jugs or other flotation devices at arm's length (which can strain your back, shoulder, neck, and elbow joints). When using jugs, hold them firmly under your arms with open palms around the jug handles. Grasping the handles too firmly can elevate the blood pressure or aggravate arthritis in your hands. Those who are not comfortable with jugs (people with shoulder injuries, arthritis, bursitis, or hand limitations) should use alternate flotation such as flotation belts, buoys, vests, upper-arm rings, or other appropriate flotation devices that do not force you into a forward, backward, or unstable position.

When your abdominal muscles become fatigued, they cannot protect your spine from pain-producing hyperextension. Slow, continuous exercise at a moderate speed that ends before fatigue sets in protects you from developing lower-back injury brought on by overenthusiastic abdominal exercise. In the water, many people can perform more exercises with better control, maintain more comfortable body position, and gain more strength with reduced risk of injury.

Back

In addition to abdominal muscle strengthening and flexibility conditioning for your back and your lower body, physicians' recommendations include maintaining strong back extensor muscles to ward off lower-back pain caused by muscle weakness. To strengthen these muscles gently while you are standing in the pool, begin in the flat back position shown in figure 3.3*a*, place your hands at midthigh and round your back toward the sky to form a "mountain" shape (see figure 3.3*b*). Then return to a flat back position, continually supporting your weight, with your hands on your thighs. For improved back flexibility and strength, repeat slowly the exercise illustrated in figures 3.3*a* and *b* several times and finish with a 20-second static stretch in the position shown in figure 3.3*b*.

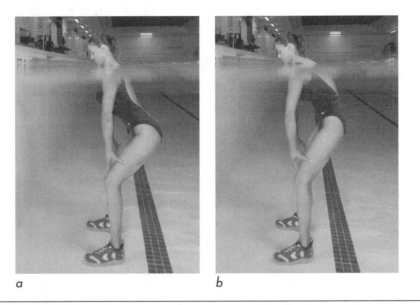

a   b

Figure 3.3   Back extensions: Begin in *(a)* the flat position and *(b)* round your back into a mountain shape.

Exercise Precautions   Every body is different and the back is no exception. When people push too far or too soon, the back is often the first area to suffer. With back exercises, as with all exercises, work within your controllable range of motion and never push past pain. Pain is a signal to stop or change what you are doing to accommodate your current fitness level, refine your biomechanics, or adjust your stabilization posture.

Upper Body

Balanced strength in the upper torso muscles (figure 3.4) can help prevent or correct postural problems such as rounded shoulders or neck pain. Water exercise balances and strengthens your shoulders, chest, and upper back by working your body against resistance in both directions during the same exercise. The complete exercise program illustrated in chapter 6, Strengthening and Toning, provides a sequence that conditions your upper-body muscles for the purpose of developing healthy, balanced musculature.

Start without disks or resistance and then gradually increase the degree of intensity by adding resistance equipment; start at slower speeds and build as you become stronger.

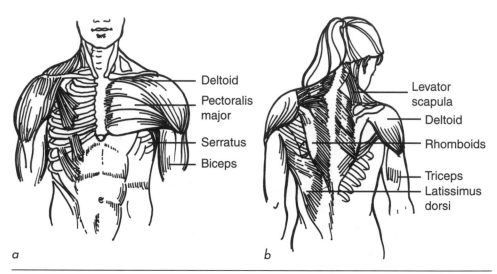

a   b

Figure 3.4 The muscles of the upper body from the *(a)* front and *(b)* back.

Exercise Precautions   Maintain a stable position, with your feet planted firmly on the bottom of the pool and your body aligned in the neutral position (figure 3.5a). Be sure to keep your shoulder blades down and back; this position stimulates and conditions the stabilizer muscles to do a better job and represents an essential element of building core strength. The muscles of the torso work as stabilizers during upper-body exercises and during most day-to-day tasks. As you become stronger, you can march in place to stay warm. Avoid hyperextending your lower back (figure 3.5b).

Lower Body

Familiarize yourself with the anatomy of your lower body (figure 3.6). Although improvements in appearance aid in motivation, the real objective is strength in your knee, hip, and lower back. Aerobic exercise reduces the fat storage in your body. Healthy appearance, attractive posture, and enhanced injury prevention come along with conditioned, balanced muscles. Work the thighs, buttocks, and hips in all directions—front, back, and sides—using the Front Leg Kick, Back Knee Curl, and Side Lunge Step. Strengthen and tone your thighs, hips, buttocks, and back with the Knee Lift, Press-Back, and Side Leg Lift. Perform the Water Squat to enhance your torso, knees, back, buttocks, and thighs and include the Water Squat in movement combinations to work your entire lower body in unison effectively.

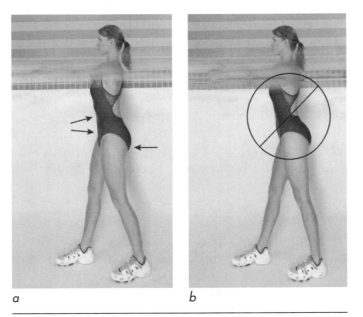

a   b

Figure 3.5 Begin in (a) the braced neutral position with one leg forward and one leg back, contracting the abdominals and buttocks. Avoid (b) lumbar spine hyperextension.

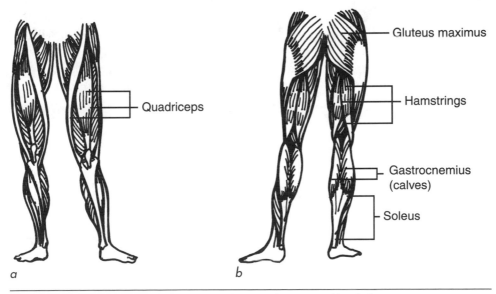

a   b

Figure 3.6 The muscles of the lower body from the front (a) and back (b).

To improve strength in your shins, walk on your heels or tap your toes to work the front of your lower leg. Most of the aerobic exercises you perform in shallow water work your calf, so you need to strengthen your shins to keep the muscles in balance and prevent injury.

See chapter 6, Strengthening and Toning, for specifics on exercises to strengthen and tone your lower body.

Exercise Precautions   Focus on protecting your back during lower-body exercise by using strong abdominal muscle control and maintaining firm pelvic neutral posture: To ensure back safety and improve core strength, brace your pelvis in the neutral position and contract your abdominal and buttocks muscles throughout each exercise. Avoid hyperextending your lower back by jutting out your stomach and curving your lower back. To protect your upper spine and neck, keep your shoulder blades back and down. Move at a speed that allows you to perform each exercise in complete control, without losing your stabilized positioning.

Cool-Down and Stretch

Warm muscles respond well to flexibility exercises. The stretches performed at the end of your exercise routine are designed to maintain or increase flexibility around your body joints. During the final stretch, maintain static, steady stretch positions for 10 to 20 seconds each to let the muscle completely relax and cool in its fully lengthened position. Adequate flexibility is the key for preventing injury. However, more is not better; stretching should never hurt.

Exercise Precautions   Hold the position and stretch to the point of comfortable resistance but no pain. Bouncing a stretch produces microscopic tears in the muscle and can actually cause the muscle to shorten. Follow the stretch instructions carefully to be sure that you are in the proper position, with all of your joints protected. Everyone exhibits differing degrees of flexibility, so avoid comparing yourself to someone else. Do what feels comfortable for you. You may be more flexible on some days than others, so listen to your body and adjust the degree of stretch according to how you feel that day.

CHAPTER 4

Warming Up and Cooling Down

Warm up and cool down to improve flexibility. Flexible muscles and tendons are extremely important in the prevention of strain or sprain injuries. When muscles and tendons are flexible and supple, they can move and perform without being overstretched. However, if your muscles and tendons are tight and stiff, you can easily push them beyond their range of motion. When that happens, strains, sprains, and pulled muscles result. To keep your muscles and tendons flexible and supple, it is important to undertake a structured stretching routine that you maintain on a regular basis, most days of the week.

Thermal Warm-Up and Stretch

Prepare your body for more challenging exercise by starting with a mild, rhythmic warm-up that progresses gradually, in order to increase blood flow and warm your muscles before stretching. Engage in rhythmic warm-up moves and let the refreshing environment of the pool wake up your senses and stimulate enthusiasm. Then complete a thorough and properly performed stretch routine to lengthen your muscles and ready your tendons prior to beginning aerobic and muscle toning activity. This warm-up can prevent injury and reduce the incidence or degree of soreness. Without a proper warm-up and stretch sequence, your muscles and tendons remain tight and stiff. Blood flow to the areas around your joints and back may be limited, which results in a lack of oxygen and nutrients for your muscles—a recipe for muscle or tendon injury.

Before any activity, be sure to warm up thoroughly and stretch all of the muscles and tendons that you will use during the activity. Following your workout, rest and recovery are extremely important, especially for athletes or for anyone whose lifestyle involves strenuous physical activity. Be sure to let your muscles rest and recover after vigorous workouts.

Perform the Thermal Warm-Up and Stretch exercises in numerical order at the beginning of every workout session. For best results, include all of the stretches listed, although you can warm up with any light rhythmic movement that does not elevate your heart rate toward your peak aerobic target zone. The Warm-Up and Stretch sequence takes about 10 minutes to complete. Begin in waist- to chest-deep water. Throughout the warm-up and the entire water workout, concentrate on stabilizing or bracing your spine in the neutral position by contracting your abdominals and buttocks. In instances in which stabilizing your spine is particularly important, the reminder is repeated. Most individuals should avoid use of resistive equipment during the Thermal Warm-Up. For additional safety and success tips, refer to the Injury Prevention Checklist in Chapter 2, Preparing for Water Workouts.

Thermal Warm-Up Moves (5 minutes)

To begin the Thermal Warm-Up, enter the water and start moving. The sooner you begin moving, the more quickly you feel comfortable in the water. Being in the water often makes people feel cool because the water dissipates heat from the skin and movement warms the blood and tissues. Use smooth, flowing motions to warm up; give your body a chance to acclimate to the water environment by sending blood, fluids, oxygen, and nutrients circulating to the working muscles and by lubricating the joints. Perform each rhythmic move in order or distribute and repeat them throughout the Thermal Warm-Up for more variation. Be sure to start with striding; give your body ample opportunity to acclimate to movement in the viscous (more resistant) environment of water and then shift continuously from one move to the next. After you have warmed up rhythmically for 5 to 10 minutes, your muscles and joints are ready for Warm-Up Stretches.

WATER WALK

Starting Position: Stand upright, with your abdominal muscles firm and your buttocks contracted in order to brace your pelvic spine in a neutral position. Keep your shoulder blades down and back and your chest lifted.

Action:

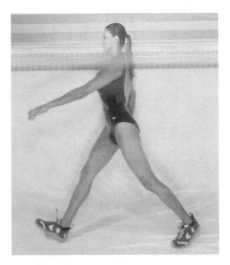

1. Stride or jog forward 8 steps, then back 4 steps.

2. Stay upright and maintain the stabilized neutral pelvic position throughout the exercise.

3. Slide relatively straight arms forward and back at your sides as you walk.

4. Use your arms in opposition to your legs: When you step forward with your right leg, slide your left arm forward and vice versa, palms facing your thighs. Most people need to practice this movement for awhile before it becomes natural. This technique not only strengthens and tones muscles, but the action of synchronizing the alternate arms and legs keeps your torso upright while building improvements in your posture, balance, and coordination.

5. Continue striding for several minutes until you are ready to switch to another move.

Variations:

- Walk forward and backward with short steps, long steps, average steps, or step kicks.
- Move in the pattern of a circle or square.

When you are ready to increase intensity,

- stride by taking very large controlled steps, and
- bound by pushing off with your back foot to bounce up off the pool floor between strides.

Safety Tips: When circling, be sure to turn around midway and circle in the other direction to balance the physical demands on your body. Even when you are warming up, postural alignment is very important. Lift up through the crown of your head and bring your shoulder blades back and down. Brace your hips and pelvis in a neutral position at the pelvis by contracting your abdominal muscles and squeezing your buttocks. As you stride, concentrate on maintaining this body alignment to protect and strengthen the muscles that protect your spine and prevent back and neck pain.

PEDAL JOG

Starting Position: Get into a jogging ready position. Stand upright, with your abdominal muscles firm and your buttocks contracted in order to brace your pelvic spine in a neutral position. Keep your shoulder blades down and back and your chest lifted.

Action:

1. Instead of lifting your whole foot from the floor as you would when running, alternately lift one heel and then the other.

2. Pump your arms up and down or back and forth in opposition to your legs.

3. Continue to pedal jog until you are ready to move on to another warm-up action.

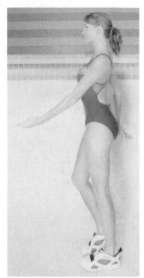

Safety Tips: Lift up through the crown of your head, and bring your shoulder blades back and down. Brace your hips and pelvis in a neutral position at the pelvis by contracting your abdominal muscles and squeezing your buttocks.

POMP AND CIRCUMSTANCE

Starting Position: Stand upright, with your abdominal muscles firm and your buttocks contracted in order to brace your pelvic spine in a neutral position. Keep your shoulder blades down and back and your chest lifted.

Action:

1. Walk as you would during a formal procession during graduation in exaggerated, large steps. Take one long step forward with your right leg. Swing your opposite arm forward from the shoulder, slicing the water with your hand, palm facing your side or cupped to catch the water. Keep your hands under the surface of the water during the movements.

2. Step together: Bring your left foot forward to meet your right foot. Return your arm to your side.

3. Take one long step forward with your left leg. Swing your opposite arm forward from the shoulder, the palm facing your side or cupped.

4. Step together: Bring your right foot forward to meet your left foot. Return your arm to your side.

5. Perform the same exercise backward to cross the pool in the opposite direction. Repeat, moving forward 8 steps and back 8 steps.

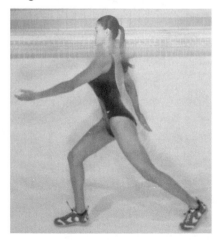

KNEE-LIFT JOG OR MARCH

Starting Position: Stand upright, with your abdominal muscles firm and your buttocks contracted in order to brace your pelvic spine in a neutral position. Keep your shoulder blades down and back and your chest lifted.

Action: Alternately lift one knee and then the other, moving your arms and legs in opposition to one another to elevate your body response and increase your body temperature.

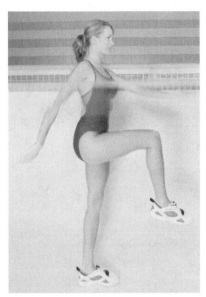

1. Lift your right knee as you press your opposite arm forward from the shoulder; keep your elbow slightly bent, slicing the water with your hand, with your palm facing your side or cupping the water.

2. Put your foot down and bring your arm back to your side.

3. Lift your left knee as you press your opposite arm forward from the shoulder; keep your elbow bent, slicing the water with your hand, with your palm facing your side or cupping the water.

4. Put your foot down and bring your arm back to your side.

Variations:

- Jog: Jog in place, hopping from foot to foot as you lift your knees.
- March: Push off the bottom of the pool to build intensity. Avoid the push-off hop if your goal is to reduce intensity or impact shock. As you become more fit, build intensity gradually, starting with low lifts or slow lifts and then building to "double time" and lifting your knees as high as feels comfortable and controllable.

Safety Tips: Keep your pelvic posture aligned in neutral by bracing your spine between contracted abdominals and buttocks to protect your lower back. Avoid lifting your knees beyond hip height. Start with your legs first and add your arms later, when you have mastered the legs.

TOY SOLDIER MARCH

Starting Position: Stand upright, with your abdominal muscles firm and your buttocks contracted in order to brace your pelvic spine in a neutral position. Keep your shoulder blades down and back and your chest lifted.

Action:

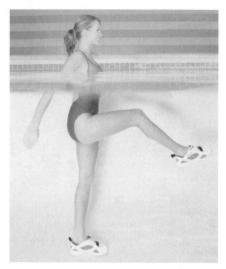

1. Firm up your abdominal muscle contraction. Lift your right leg from the hip; keep your knee straight. At the same time, reach forward from the shoulder with your left arm, with a slight bend at the elbow, slicing the water with your hand. Lift your leg only as high as is comfortable for you and maintain postural stability. Put your leg down as you bring your arm to your side.

2. Lift your left leg from the hip; keep your knee straight. At the same time, reach forward from the shoulder with your right arm with a slight bend at the elbow. Put your leg down (moving from the hip) and bring your arm to your side.

3. March with straight legs.

Safety Tips: Start with your legs first and add your arms later, when you have mastered the legs. Keep your pelvis aligned by bracing your spine between contracted abdominal and buttocks muscles. Avoid hyperextending (over-straightening) at the knee.

CAN-CAN KICK

Starting Position: Stand upright. Brace the position of your spine in neutral at the pelvis by contracting your abdominal and buttocks muscles. Keep your chest lifted. Open your chest by keeping your shoulder blades back and down with your abdominal muscles firm and your buttocks contracted in order to brace your pelvic spine in a neutral position.

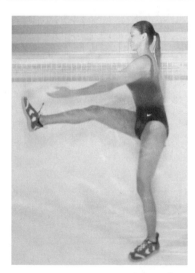

Action:

1. Kick your right leg forward, contracting your abdominals as you lift your leg from your hip, like a football punter. At the same time, swing your opposite arm forward from your shoulder. Maintain a slight bend at your knee.

2. As you lower your right leg, hop onto your right foot and kick your left leg forward, lifting your leg from your hip. As you swing the right arm forward from your shoulder, lower your left arm to your side. Maintain a slight bend at your knee. Determine the height of the kick based on what is most comfortable for you. Kick only as high as you can while still maintaining proper body alignment. Keep all of your kicks below hip height.

3. Alternate kicks for 8 to 16 repetitions.

Safety Tip: If you have ever experienced chronic back pain, keep your kicks extra low.

KICK UP YOUR HEELS

MOVE
7

Starting Position: Stand with your feet about shoulder-width apart.

Action:

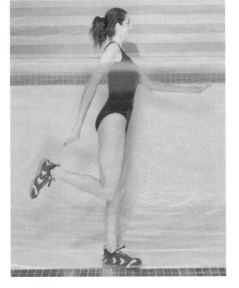

1. Contract (tighten) your ab-dominal muscles to protect your spine. Open your chest by bringing your shoulder blades back and down. Maintain this stabilization throughout the exercise.

2. Cup your hand and scoop forward with your left arm as you lift your right heel toward your buttocks, keeping your thighs parallel to each other and perpendicular to the floor.

3. Return your arm and leg to standing position.

4. Brace your torso position. Cup your hand and scoop forward with your right arm as you lift your left heel toward your buttocks, keeping your thighs parallel to each other and perpendicular to the floor.

5. Return your arms and legs to starting position.

6. Repeat 16 times.

Variation: To increase intensity, do the exercise without placing one foot down before lifting the other; instead, jump from foot to foot as you kick up each heel.

SIDE KNEE HOP

Starting Position: Stand with your feet shoulder-width apart and your arms out in front of your chest, palms facing outward with thumbs down. Stabilize your torso by contracting your abdominals and buttocks and keeping your shoulder blades back and down.

Action:

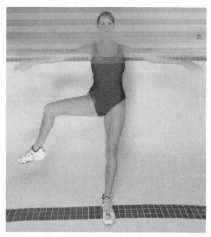

1. Hop and lift your right knee up and out to the right while you press your hands out to either side.

2. Hop and bring your feet together, putting your foot back on the floor. At the same time, press your hands toward one another, with your arms outstretched in front of your chest.

3. Hop and lift your left knee up and out to the side while you press your palms out to either side.

4. Hop and bring your feet together, putting your foot back down on the floor. At the same time, press your hands toward one another, with your arms outstretched in front of your chest.

5. Repeat 8 to 16 times.

Variation: Eliminate the small hop between movements to reduce the intensity or the impact shock of this exercise.

Safety Tips: Work extra hard to keep your shoulders down and back on this exercise in order to prevent neck pain. To protect and strengthen your back, be sure to brace your pelvis in a neutral position by contracting your abdominals and buttocks.

HEEL JACKS

Starting Position: Begin with your hands at your sides, feet together. Stabilize your torso by contracting abdominal and buttocks muscles and keeping the shoulder blades down and back. Heel Jacks are similar to Jumping Jacks.

Action:

1. Coil up slightly, push off the bottom of the pool, and then jump up and press your right heel out to the side at whatever distance still allows you to place your heel on the pool floor. At the same time, press both hands outward from your sides, palms facing out. Keep a slight bend at the knee.

2. Coil slightly, jump up and bring both feet back together and press your hands toward your sides, palms facing in.

3. Jump up and press your left heel out to the side and place it on the pool floor. Press both hands outward from your sides, palms facing out. Keep a slight bend at the knee.

4. Jump up and bring both feet back together and press your hands toward your sides, palms facing in.

5. Repeat 8 to 16 times.

Variation: Add a small hop onto both feet at once between each movement to heighten the intensity and fun of this exercise.

Safety Tips: Land with slightly bent knees. Special attention to contraction of the abdominals on each jump protects and strengthens your back.

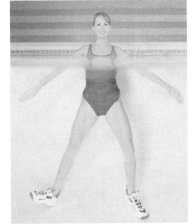

ALTERNATE LEG PRESS-BACK

Starting Position: Start with your feet together and your arms at your sides. Contract (tighten) your abdominal and buttocks muscles to avoid hyperextending (curving) at your lower back as you press your leg backward. The movement performed in Alternate Leg Press-Back is similar to a lunge.

Action:

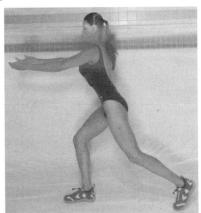

1. Press both arms straight out in front, scooping your arms forward, palms first. At the same time, lift your left knee; then, from the hips, press your left foot all the way back, touching your toes on the pool floor behind you. Your right knee bends.

2. Bring both feet back together again and then scoop your palms back toward your sides.

3. Again, press both arms straight out in front, scooping forward with your palms as you lift your right knee; then, from the hips, press your right foot all the way back, touching your toes on the pool floor behind you. Bend left knee.

4. Bring both feet back together again and scoop your palms back toward your sides. Breathe deeply.

5. Repeat sequence 8 to 16 times.

Variation: Add a small hop between movements to increase the intensity of this exercise. If you are prone to knee or back pain or seek greater stability, eliminate the bounce and perform this exercise facing the pool wall or ladder and hold on with both hands. Use this exercise to build your torso and knee stability while you are supported by the wall or ladder.

Safety Tips: Concentrate on keeping your front knee over your heel rather than over your toes. Bracing your pelvis firmly in a neutral position by contracting your abdominal and buttocks muscles helps prevent back pain and strengthens your postural muscles.

MOVE
11

KNEE-LIFT KICK

Starting Position: Begin with your feet shoulder-width apart, hands at your sides. Tighten your abdominals and squeeze your buttocks to brace your spine.

Action:

1. Lift your left knee toward your chest, no higher than hip height. At the same time, reach your opposite arm forward from the shoulder (figure *a*).
2. Then kick your left leg forward from the knee. Kick only as high as is comfortable for you, to a height that does not pull you out of braced neutral position at the pelvis (figure *b*).
3. Bend your knee, then return your foot to the floor of the pool, and bring your arm to your side.
4. Repeat the sequence with your right leg and left arm.
5. Repeat the sequence 8 times.

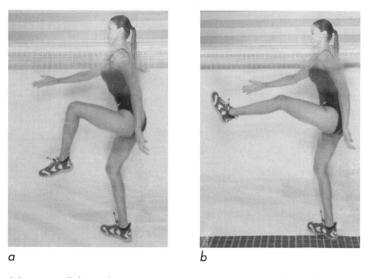

a   b

Variation: Add a small hop between movements to increase the intensity of this exercise.

Safety Tips: As you kick forward, be sure to maintain a slight bend at your knee to eliminate hyperextension. Keep your abdominals contracted to avoid dipping your pelvis forward and under during the kick phase. In other words, keep your torso lifted up straight and firm.

Thermal Warm-Up Stretches (5 minutes)

Stretching Technique: Stretch each major muscle group carefully to prepare your body for exercise and to prevent injury. The instructions are designed to move you smoothly and continuously from stretch to stretch in the order listed. As you become more familiar with the stretches, you may change the sequence to add variety, but be sure to stretch the muscle group near to the one you just finished stretching to help prevent muscle tears.

During Warm-Up Stretches, hold each static stretch position for 10 seconds (avoid bouncing, which causes a reflexive shortening of the muscle). At the end of your workout, hold each Final Cool-Down Stretch for 20 seconds. Remember to stretch only to the point where you feel a comfortable degree of resistance. If you feel pain or discomfort, you are either stretching too far (ease up on the stretch and allow your muscles to relax) or you are out of position (double check the instructions and illustrations).

Because water cools the body quickly, you can continuously move your arms through the water while stretching your lower body to keep your muscles supple and your body comfortably warm. But if your shoulder joints are tender or vulnerable, you may want to minimize such arm movements during stretching. You can also march or pedal jog in place to stay warm while you stretch your upper body if you are able to keep your stretch and torso position stable while doing so.

Lower Body

Perform the first nine stretches at pool side (Outer-Thigh Stretch through Hamstring Stretch). Complete all nine stretches while holding on to the pool edge or ladder with your left hand unless instructed otherwise. Then turn around and complete the same stretches for the other side of your body while holding on with your right hand.

OUTER-THIGH STRETCH

STRETCH
1

Starting Position: Stand with your right side toward the pool wall, holding on to the pool edge with your right hand.

Action:

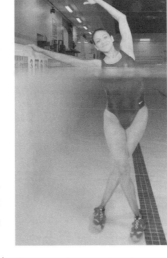

1. Stand up straight and cross your outside leg over the leg nearest to the side of the pool.
2. Reach up with your free arm and lean your hip away from the pool edge.

Variation: With your free arm, scoop your palm toward the wall. Then turn your palm around and press away from the wall. Repeat this arm action slowly, in time to the music if you are using it.

Relax the muscles on the outside of your left thigh and hold the stretch position, without bouncing, for approximately 10 seconds or for about 16 beats of the music (10 seconds for Warm-Up Stretches; 20 seconds for Cool-Down Stretches).

Safety Tips: Keep both of your shoulders relaxed. Be sure to contract your abdominals firmly and keep both hips facing forward (avoid twisting) so that the position doesn't put strain on your lower back. Breathe deeply to encourage your muscles to relax.

2 LOWER-BACK STRETCH WITH ANKLE ROTATION

Starting Position: Hold on to the pool edge. Stand up straight and firmly contract your abdominal muscles.

Action:

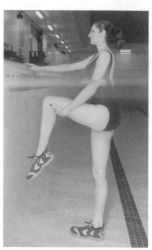

1. Lift your left leg. Reach under your thigh as you draw your knee toward your chest, and relax your lower back.
2. Slowly roll your foot in a counterclockwise circle for several revolutions. Then roll it clockwise. Rotate your ankle through your full range of motion. (Roll it in as wide a circle as possible without causing pain.)
3. Repeat with your right leg.

Safety Tip: Stand upright with your chest lifted and your shoulder blades back and down.

3 FRONT-OF-THIGH STRETCH

Starting Position: Turn your back to the wall and stand about 18 inches (.5 m) from it. Reach back and hold on to the pool edge with your outstretched right arm and place your left foot on the wall behind you.

Action:

1. Standing up straight, squeeze your abdominal muscles in tight and push your hips away from the wall so that your knee joint forms a right angle.
2. Breathe deeply and relax the front of your thigh.

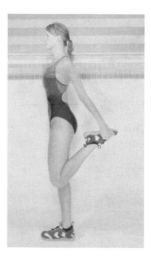

Variation: If it is comfortable and you can perform this without arching your back, reach for your foot and bring it toward your buttocks as you point your knee straight down. Both thighs should be parallel and perpendicular to the floor.

Safety Tip: Be sure to pull in your abdominals and contract your buttocks slightly to keep your spine aligned in pelvic neutral.

SHIN STRETCH AND SHOULDER SHRUG

Starting Position: Turn your body so that you are standing with your right side toward the pool wall.

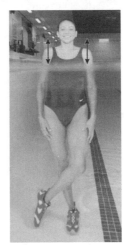

Action:

1. Cross your outside leg over your inside leg. Point your foot and place the tops of your toes on the floor of the pool. Breathe deeply and relax your shin.

2. While you stretch your shin, slowly raise both shoulders toward your ears; then slowly depress your shoulders. Keep your chest open and your shoulders back. Repeat the movement slowly in time to the music.

Safety Tip: If coordinating both the Shin Stretch and the Shoulder Shrug at the same time throws you off balance, perform each movement separately.

INNER-THIGH STEP-OUT

Starting Position: Stand with both feet on the floor, with your right side toward the pool wall.

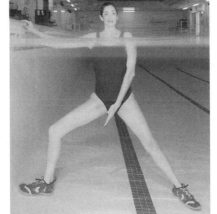

Action: Step out to the side, bending your right knee and moving your left leg as far from your torso as you find comfortable. Relax your inner thigh, hold a steady, nonbouncing stretch, and breathe deeply.

Variation: To stay warm, press your palm toward and then away from the pool wall in time to the music.

Safety Tips: Keep your bent knee positioned over your heel to prevent undue pressure at your knee joint. If your knee is pushing out over your toes, place your feet wider apart.

6 | HIP FLEXOR STRETCH

Starting Position: Hold on to the pool edge. Stand with one foot in front and place the other foot back behind you at a comfortable distance.

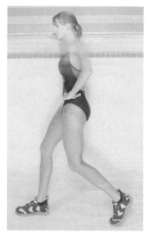

Action:

1. With your front knee bent, straighten your back leg and raise your back heel (you are on the toes of your back foot).

2. Pull in your abdominal muscles and gently press your hips down and forward to stretch the hip flexor muscles that run from your torso to the front of your thigh.

Variation: With your free hand (the one not holding the pool edge), press your palm toward and then away from the pool wall in time to the music.

Safety Tips: Keep your bent knee positioned over your heel to prevent undue pressure at your knee joint. Place your feet wider apart from front to back if your front knee is pushing out over your toes or if you don't feel a stretch at the hip flexor.

7 | STRAIGHT-LEG CALF STRETCH

Starting Position: After the Hip Flexor Stretch, you are standing with one foot in front of the other. Move your back foot a bit closer to your front foot. The distance apart is determined by your degree of flexibility: Look at your back foot; you should be able to point your toes straight ahead. If you can't, shorten the distance between your front foot and your back foot.

Action:

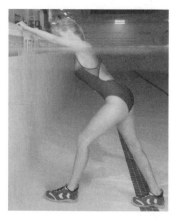

1. Press your heel down to the floor. Be sure that your back foot is pointing straight ahead and that your front knee is over your heel rather than over your toes.

2. Relax your calf muscle at the back of your lower leg.

Variation: Press your free arm toward and then away from the pool wall in time to the music.

Safety Tips: If your calf muscle feels tight and uncomfortable or if you have difficulty relaxing your calf muscle, bring your back foot a little closer to your front foot until you can press your heel to the floor comfortably. Look back and make sure that your back foot points straight ahead, not out to the side. When calf muscles are tight, you may tend to splay your foot out to the side. To perform this stretch properly, make sure that your hips are equal distance from the pool wall, and your back foot is pointed straight ahead.

BENT-KNEE CALF STRETCH

Starting Position: Stand with one foot in front of the other, in the position for the Straight-Leg Calf Stretch.

Action:

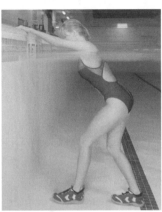

1. Bring your back foot another step closer to your front foot.
2. Bend both knees.
3. Continue to support your weight on your front leg. Relax your calf muscle and Achilles tendon.

Variation: Press one palm toward and then away from the pool wall in time to the music.

Safety Tips: Be sure to complete both the Straight-Leg Calf Stretch and the Bent-Knee Calf Stretch. Both stretches are necessary because of the structural makeup of your lower leg. The second calf stretch helps prevent Achilles tendonitis, and both stretches help keep your foot as well as your calf flexible. Keep your abdominals and buttocks contracted firmly to brace the position of your spine.

HAMSTRING STRETCH

Starting Position: Face the pool wall.

Action:

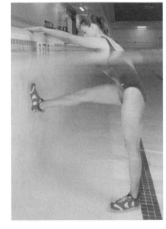

1. Place your right foot against the wall at a height that allows you to straighten your leg comfortably without locking or hyperextending your knee.
2. Pull in your abdominals, keep your back flat, and lean forward from your hip. Relax and soften the muscles at the back of your thigh.
3. Hold on to the pool edge for stability.

Safety Tips: Keep a very slight bend at the knee of the leg that you are stretching. Avoid overstraightening, which is called hyperextension. Flatten your back, rather than rounding it, to ensure that the hamstring receives a proper stretch.

Back

Flexible lower-body muscles help prevent, ease, or eliminate lower-back pain. Here are three more stretches to encourage a healthy back.

STRETCH 10   DEEP-MUSCLE HIP, THIGH, AND BUTTOCKS STRETCH

Starting Position: Face the pool wall, with both hands on the edge.

Action:

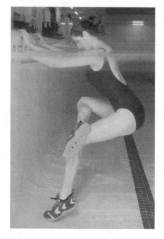

1. Cross your right ankle at your left knee and slowly lower yourself as if you were sitting in a chair.
2. Relax your buttocks, hip, and outer thigh; contract your abdominal muscles; and breathe deeply.
3. Hold the stretch for 10 seconds (warm-up) or 20 seconds (cool-down).
4. Put both feet on the floor and stand up; then repeat the stretch with your left ankle at your right knee.

Safety Tips: Be sure to keep your back flat as you lean forward from your hips. Stretch only as far as you feel a comfortable amount of resistance; then focus on relaxing the muscles of your buttocks, lower back, and thigh. To enhance the stretch, breathe deeply into the stretch and release muscle tension as you exhale.

STRETCH 11   FULL BACK STRETCH

Starting Position: Continue facing the pool wall, with both hands holding onto the edge.

Action:

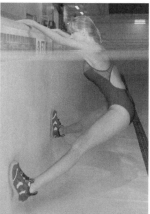

1. Lower yourself into the water and place your feet more than shoulder-width apart against the wall. The water buoys your body.
2. Relax and soften the muscles of your entire back.

Safety Tips: Lean forward from your hips with a straight back to enhance the stretch. If you do not have a ledge that allows you to hold on comfortably without slipping, perform this stretch at the pool ladder.

MIDBACK STRETCH

Starting Position: Stand in waist- to chest-deep water, with your feet more than shoulder-width apart and your knees bent and over your heels. Stand near the edge of the pool, with your side toward the pool wall.

Action:

1. To support your body weight, place both hands on the tops of your thighs, midway between hip and knee. Lean forward and look at the bottom of the pool (figure *a*). Take a deep breath and then exhale and arch your back upward toward the sky as you contract your abdominals and buttocks. Breathing deeply, hold the position for 10 seconds and relax your back (20 seconds for Cool-Down Stretch). Then press yourself up slowly with your hands on your thighs to prevent stress to your lower back, rising one vertebra at a time.

2. Keep your knees bent. Reach both hands toward the wall and lightly grasp the pool edge with both hands (or place one hand on the arm closest to the wall if this is too far to stretch) (figure *b*). Breathe fully and evenly as you hold the position for 10 seconds and soften the muscles of your back (20 seconds for Cool-Down Stretch). Be sure to keep your hips facing straight ahead, not twisted toward the pool wall.

3. Bring your feet closer together, about shoulder-width apart. Reach both hands toward the wall and grasp the pool edge with both hands (or place one hand on the arm closest to the wall if this is too far to stretch). Breathe fully and evenly as you hold the position for 10 seconds and soften the muscles of your back (20 seconds for Cool-Down Stretch). Be sure to keep your hips facing straight ahead, not twisted toward the pool wall.

4. Turn around and repeat steps 1 through 3.

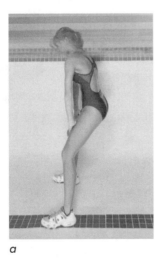
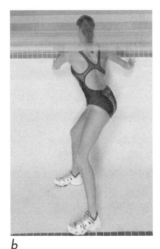

a   *b*

Safety Tips: Never push a stretch beyond the comfortable range of motion. This is particularly important with a stretch such as the Midback Stretch that requires a slight twist. Listen to your body to feel how far it is ready to stretch.

Upper Body

Step away from the wall and perform these additional upper-body stretches.

STRETCH 13   ELBOW PRESS-BACK

Starting Position: Stand in the neutral position, with your feet shoulder-width apart. Place your hands behind your head, with your fingertips gently planted at the base of your skull and your elbows in front.

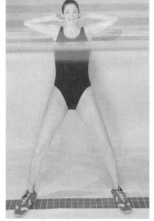

Action:

1. Perform this exercise very slowly: Press both elbows back as you squeeze the muscles of your shoulder blades together and down and take a deep breath.
2. Exhale slowly as you bring your elbows toward each other.
3. Repeat 4 to 8 times.

Safety Tips: Avoid pressing your head forward as you press your elbows back. With each repetition, contract your abdominal muscles more firmly to protect your lower back.

STRETCH 14   SHOULDER ROLL AND CHEST STRETCH

Starting Position: Stand in the neutral position, with your feet shoulder-width apart.

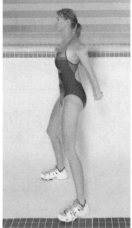

Action:

1. Raise both shoulders up toward your ears. Roll your shoulders backward as you bring your shoulder blades together. Then lower your shoulders and roll them forward. Repeat 8 to 16 times.
2. Contract your abdomen and roll your shoulders back. Bring both hands backward, clasp them behind your back, and gently open up and stretch your chest. Breathe deeply and hold the stretch for 10 seconds (20 seconds for Cool-Down Stretch).

Safety Tip: Keep your shoulders down while clasping your hands behind your back.

CHEST STRETCH

Starting Position: Stand facing the pool wall, preferably in shoulder-depth water.

Action:

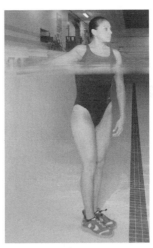

1. Raise your right arm to the right and place your palm on the pool wall at shoulder height or as high as you can at the depth available to you.
2. Turn your torso to the left slowly until you feel a comfortable amount of resistance at the muscles of your chest. Hold the position for 10 seconds for warm-up and 20 seconds for cool-down.
3. Repeat with your left arm.
4. You can perform this stretch with your palm on the wall at various heights to get a slightly different stretch for the muscles of your chest.

Safety Tips: To avoid arching your back, maintain contracted abdominal muscles. Be sure to avoid twisting your torso; turn your whole body as one piece, not just your upper body.

UPPER-BACK STRETCH

Starting Position: Stand in the neutral position, with your feet shoulder-width apart.

Action:

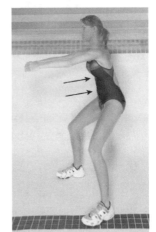

1. Bring your arms forward, reach out in front of your chest, and link your thumbs.
2. While standing up straight, contract your abdominal muscles, round your upper back, and look down at the floor of the pool.
3. Relax the muscles of your upper back, neck, and shoulders.
4. Hold for 10 seconds (20 seconds for Cool-Down Stretch).

Safety Tips: Keep your torso upright at the waist and isolate the stretch in your upper back. Keep your shoulders down.

17 TORSO AND SHOULDER STRETCH

Starting Position: Stand in the neutral position, with your feet shoulder-width apart.

Action:

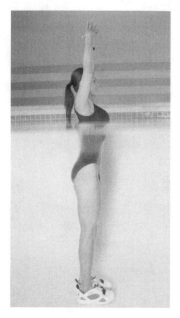

1. Contract your abdominal and buttocks muscles to stabilize your spine.
2. Bring your arms out to the sides.
3. Raise your arms overhead and link your thumbs together.
4. Lift your chest as you reach toward the sky.
5. Flex your knees slightly; lift through your torso as you bring your upper arms next to your ears, being careful not to arch your back or drop your head.
6. Breathe deeply and hold the stretch for 16 counts.

Safety Tips: Keep your elbows slightly bent to avoid stressing your elbow joint. Keep your shoulder blades down and back. If your shoulder feels tight, lower your hands in front of your face until the tightness disappears. Aim to hold your ears over your shoulders and your shoulders over your hips.

18 SHOULDER AND UPPER-ARM STRETCH

Starting Position: Stand in the neutral position, with your feet shoulder-width apart.

Action:

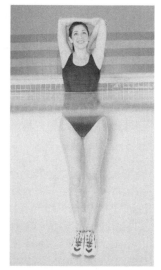

1. Reach behind your neck with your left hand.
2. Clasp your left elbow with your right hand. Draw your left elbow toward your head, just to the point of comfortable resistance. Relax your shoulder and upper arm. Keep your head up straight to protect your neck.
3. Extend your left arm.
4. Repeat the sequence with your right arm to stretch the other side.

Safety Tips: Avoid tipping your head forward. Change the position of your supporting arm (bring it in front of your face) if your head is being forced forward.

SAFE NECK STRETCH

Starting Position: Stand in the neutral position with your feet shoulder-width apart.

Action:

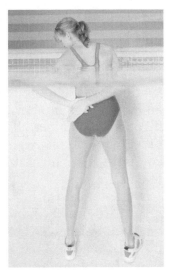

1. Reach behind your back and bring your right arm toward your left hip. Gently grasp your right wrist with your left hand. Slowly lower your left ear toward your left shoulder. Hold the stretch for 20 seconds; then return your head to an upright position. Repeat the stretch on the opposite side.

2. Reach behind your back and bring your right arm toward your left hip. Gently grasp your right wrist with your left hand. Slowly turn your head so that you are looking toward your left shoulder. Hold the stretch for 10 to 20 seconds; then turn your head slowly forward. Repeat the stretch for the opposite side.

Safety Tips: Remember to stretch only to the point of comfortable resistance. If you feel pulling or pain, you are stretching too far. Slowly reduce the amount of stretch. Move very slowly from one position to the next to avoid injury.

Final Cool-Down and Cool-Down Stretch Sequence

At the end of your workout, perform all of the stretches listed to cool your muscles in a lengthened position. Perform all of the stretches completed during warm-up, but hold each static stretch for about twice as long (20 seconds). Stretching should never be painful; stretch only to the point of comfortable resistance, and relax the muscles as you hold that position. Increase the stretch to a further degree when possible as your muscles relax. Double-check your position or eliminate the stretch temporarily if it causes discomfort. If you feel cool because you are standing relatively motionless in the water, you can stay warm by continuously moving the limbs that are not involved in the stretch.

Cool-down stretches are an excellent method to enhance and maintain flexibility: After an extended period of continuous movement, your muscles are more receptive and responsive to flexibility training. Good flexibility decreases the incidence of many types of injuries. Most people experience back pain at one time or another; chronic lower-back pain often arises from weakened abdominal muscles, combined with inadequate flexibility in the muscles of the lower body, including the back, buttocks, thigh, groin, hip flexors, and lower leg. The most common cause of lower-back pain is a job or lifestyle that involves long periods of sitting without moving or stretching, which can produce shortened torso and leg muscles and weakened abdominals.

Flexibility is determined by both heredity and physical activity, and it can vary from one part of your body to another. Stretching by cooling muscles in their lengthened position after exercise helps keep your muscles from becoming shortened, stiff, and sore. The techniques and positioning used for stretching can make or break the success of your flexibility endeavors. For instance, research suggests that people make better and safer progress by stretching muscles when they are warm. If you prefer, you can stretch a specific muscle group immediately after working it during the strengthening and toning section. Use this method to avoid becoming chilled during a segment that combines all of the stretches at the end of your routine. On the other hand, putting your stretch routine at the end of your program can help you relax and reduce stress because it allows your body to return gradually to a resting state.

Water enhances the range of motion and pain-free mobility needed for adequate flexibility training. However, be careful not to overdo flexibility training. Avoid pushing too hard, holding positions too long, or using positions that cause pain. Follow the instructions carefully to avoid improper technique. Carefully following the guidelines in the stretch diagrams minimizes the chance of injury. Stretch every day of the week as part of your regular physical activity routine.

CHAPTER 5

Benefiting From Aerobic Moves

Get lively and enjoy the unique feeling of moving about briskly in the aquatic environment. Remember to follow an aerobic progression such as the one in table 3.2 on page 44. Gradually introduce your heart, lungs, and circulatory system to the increase in exertion with an aerobic warm-up that emphasizes continuous movement using the larger muscle groups and elevates your heart rate gradually. Start with low-intensity aerobic activity (perceived exertion: fairly light). As you progress into the aerobics segment, the activity and your heart rate should build gradually to peak intensity (perceived exertion: some-what hard to hard). To prevent injury and cardiac complications, the aerobic cool-down reduces intensity gradually, allowing your cardiovascular system to return to equilibrium gradually, the way it functioned before you began aerobic exertion. By the end of the aerobic section, your heart rate should be at the low end of your target zone and your perceived exertion should be fairly light. As you move between the various segments and exercises, don't take breaks. In the water, breaks cause you to get cold. Intensity should be controlled with pace and adjusting resistance or eddy drag.

As a reminder, you can change your level of intensity in several ways.

- Vary the size of the movement: The larger the movement, the greater the water's resistance and the higher the intensity. Take larger steps to increase intensity or smaller steps to decrease intensity.

- Increase your movements to and from different locations in the pool (side to side, circle, back and forth) to elevate your heart rate. Stay in one place to lower your intensity.

- Increase or decrease speed of movement to raise or lower the amount of force needed to push your body through the water.

- Increase or decrease the surface area you are pushing through the water. For instance, cupped hands resist more water than balled fists or slices. Figure 5.1 shows the three options for hand position used to vary intensity. Keep your hands under water during all of the moves (unless otherwise indicated) to work against the water and to prevent injury caused by abrupt changes in resistance.

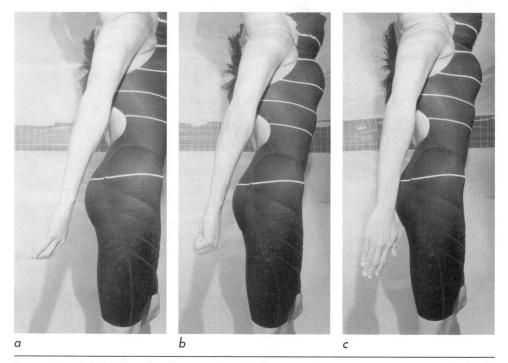

a   b   c

Figure 5.1 (a) Cup your hands to increase the intensity of resistance to your upper body. (b) Fold your hand into a fist to reduce intensity. (c) Slice your hand sideways through the water to minimize resistance.

The aerobic sequence begins with the essential warm-up and repeats the same exercises as the Thermal Warm-Up, but with the difference that it guides you to increase the intensity gradually. It then takes you through a progressive sequence to peak intensity and, finally, cools you down by returning to the exercises used in the warm-up section. Select several moves that you like and add more later for variety. In this chapter are exercises to be performed in shallow water or in deep water with flotation equipment. For more variety, add some moves from chapter 9, Adding Splash to Workouts. Chapter 7, Intensifying Workouts, provides excellent ways to advance your fitness and intensify your workout. You can tailor your workout to your specific needs by consulting chapter 8, Creating a Personal Water Workout, and chapter 10, Special Workouts for Special Needs. Older adults or individuals who have been inactive may find the Older Adult, First Water Workout, or other exercise sequences for special concerns described in chapter 10 to be more appropriate for them. For all of the workouts, practice the leg movements first; then add the arms when you feel ready. Again, avoid any move you find uncomfortable. As you become more fit, you become more proficient and comfortable with most of the exercises.

Warm-Up Aerobics

First perform the same moves as those shown in the Thermal Warm-Up (chapter 4, Warming Up and Cooling Down), but build gradually to more vigorous intensity. You can warm up simply by striding forward and back, sideways, and in circles, or you can add in as many low-intensity aerobic moves as you wish on any given day. Be sure to include an aerobic warm-up sequence that lasts for about 5 or 10 minutes before you advance into intermediate and peak aerobic intensity. Begin with Moves #1 to 11 and then continue with the additional aerobic warm-up exercises that follow: Moves #12 to 16. Pick and choose the moves that appeal to you, adding to your repertoire as you are ready to learn new moves. Be sure to warm up from front to back and side to side, moving in multiple directions.

SNAKE WALK

Starting Position: Move into waist- to chest-deep water. Pull in your abdominals and contract your buttocks firmly to brace your spine in neutral position.

Action:

1. Push your body through the water as you stride with large steps. Step forward with your left leg as you reach forward with your right arm (figure *a*). When you are just starting out, it's most important to let your arm *movement* be comfortable. Exact positioning isn't a priority. Step forward with your right leg as you reach forward with your left arm (figure *b*).

2. Stride around in a snaking "S" pattern to challenge your body in various directions and through the turbulence and eddies created by your wake. "Snake" all around the shallow end of the pool, in curving or winding patterns.

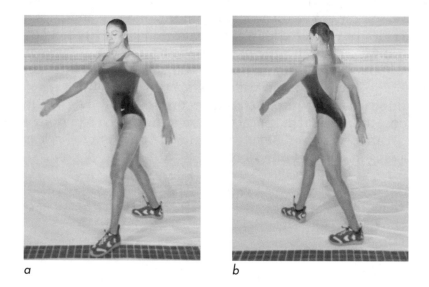

a   b

Safety Tips: Push firmly through the water, but move only as swiftly as you can manage with complete control, without weaving or losing your postural stability. Keep your head lifted, your chest open, your shoulder blades down and back, your abdominal muscles contracted, and your buttocks firm to brace your spine in neutral position.

STEP WIDE SIDE

Starting Position: Start with your feet together, arms at your sides, in waist- to chest-deep water.

Action:

1. Brace your spine and take a big step sideways with your right leg. At the same time, press your palms out to either side.

2. Then step together: Bring your left leg in to meet your right leg. Bring your palms back to your sides. Repeat this sequence, moving across the width of the pool. Then repeat the sequence, starting with the left leg, to cross the pool in the opposite direction.

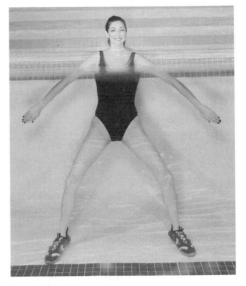

Variation: As you step together, bring your palms toward each other, but behind your back instead of to your sides. Stay lifted through your torso; avoid bending forward. This move works your shoulder differently and also gives your abdominals and core a different challenge.

Safety Tips: As you step sideways, contract your abdominals firmly to both protect your back and strengthen your core postural stabilizers. Keep your knee behind your toes and over your heel as you side step, in order to protect your knee joint.

Starting Position: Start with your feet shoulder-width apart, hands at your sides, in waist- to chest-deep water.

Action:

1. Lift your chest and brace your spine in neutral position (figure *a*); then jump up and land in a wide stance, with your knees bent and your heels down on the pool floor with your right heel pressed out to the side. Your toes should be just slightly pointed out to the sides. At the same time, press your palms out to either side. Keep your hands under the water (figure *b*).

2. Jump up and bring your feet together. Land with bent knees. At the same time, press your palms toward each other behind your buttocks.

3. Repeat the full sequence 8 times on both sides.

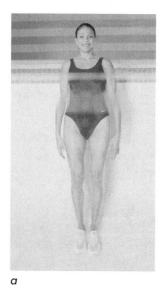
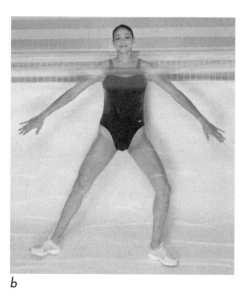

a   b

Variation: For intensified aerobic conditioning, stride or bound forward several steps and perform a Hydro Jack as you move backward with each jump.

Safety Tips: Keep your abdominals pulled in firmly and breathe deeply.

Starting Position: Stand in waist- to chest-deep water. Start with your right foot out in front of your body and your left foot back; reach with your left arm out in front (but under the water) and reach your right arm back. Determine the distance between your front and back foot based on comfort. Increase the distance between your front foot and your back foot to increase intensity.

Action:

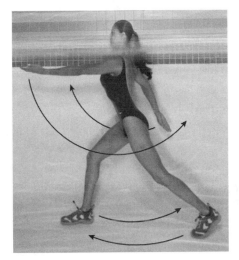

1. Lift your chest and brace your spine in neutral position. Hop up and bring your right leg forward while you press your left leg back in a cross-country ski motion. At the same time, scoop your left palm forward and press your right palm back.

2. Hop up and switch legs and arms again: Bring your left leg forward as you push your right leg back. Scoop your right palm forward as you press your left palm back.

3. Repeat for 16 sets.

Variations:

- To increase intensity, instead of skiing in place, propel your body forward and backward with the cross-country ski motion.

- To decrease intensity, shorten the distance between your front foot and back foot.

Safety Tips: Keep your front knee behind your toes, over your heel, as you land. Keep your abdominals and buttocks contracted to brace and protect your back.

MOVE 16 SAILOR'S JIG

Starting Position: Stand on your left foot, with your right leg lifted out to the side, your abdominal muscles pulled in and back braced, and both of your palms pressed sideways toward your left knee. Begin in waist- to chest-deep water.

Action: Hop from foot to foot:

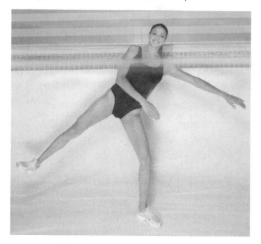

1. Hop onto your left leg as you lift your right leg out to the side. Push both palms, with your arms straight down, toward your left knee (toward the foot on which you are about to land).

2. Hop onto your right foot while you lift your left leg out to the side. Push both palms, with your arms straight down, toward your right knee.

3. Repeat for 8 sets.

Variation: For the Knee-Lift Jig, hop from foot to foot as you lift your left knee and then your right knee out to the side.

Safety Tips: Be sure to keep your shoulders down, your chest open, and your shoulder blades back in order to protect your neck and shoulders. As with any move that challenges the body core, this lateral move requires firm abdominal contraction on the side leap in order to protect your back and strengthen your core.

Peak Intensity Aerobics

Now that you have gradually increased the level of your aerobic exertion, by starting with warm-up moves and gradually building intensity, maintain your peak aerobic level by performing peak aerobics exercises. To raise your level of intensity, increase the size of the movement, travel around the pool, decrease the time it takes to travel from one end of the pool to the other, or enlarge the surface area you are pushing through water. The faster and harder you push yourself through the water and the bigger the surface area (i.e., the more viscosity your body encounters), the harder the water's resistance makes you work, raising the aerobic intensity. Use your prime mover muscle groups to propel yourself (at your hips, buttocks, legs, and shoulders), and use your stabilizer muscles to protect your joints and back (postural muscles, stabilizers in your back, neck, sides, and abdomen, especially). In the instructions for each move, pay special attention to tips on how to raise or lower intensity to suit your needs and objectives.

Important note: When raising the degree of fitness challenge, increase by only 5 to 10 percent at one time. For instance, if you have been performing 10 repetitions successfully, add one more repetition only when it is time to increase. Also, avoid increasing duration at the same time as you increase any other aspect of the *FITT principle* (Frequency, Intensity, Type, or Time).

JUMP FORWARD, JUMP BACK

MOVE
17

Starting Position: Stand in water that reaches to your rib cage or chest. Begin in the neutral position, with your spine braced; extend your arms in front, with your palms down (figure *a*).

Action:

1. Abdominal-Tuck Jump: Jump up, lifting both knees, tucking your torso, and squeezing your abdominals firmly while you press your palms backward to move forward (figure *b*).
2. Bring your feet back down, pressing your heels to the floor and bending your knees slightly.
3. Swing your arms forward, palms first, and repeat the abdominal tuck as you jump backward.

Variation: Once you have developed enough abdominal strength and corresponding level of fitness to perform Jump Forward, Jump Back without risking injury, start with 4 repetitions at moderate tempo (for example, to music with 130 beats per minute). For variety, jump forward 4 to 8 times and then backward 4 to 8 times.

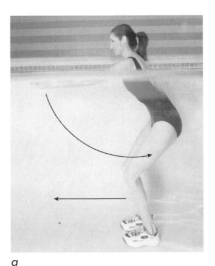

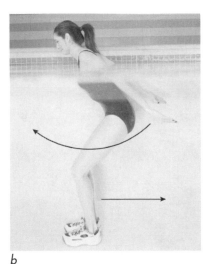

a   b

(continued)

Safety Tips: The jump requires a firm contraction of your abdominals and buttocks as well as a water power hop that incorporates the push-off training principle of plyometrics. Therefore, the Abdominal-Tuck Jump should be performed after you have gained a basic level of fitness and can control the exercise. During these exercises, your abdominal muscles work together with your back, buttocks, and hips for coordinated strength. Keep your abdominals pulled in firmly, even during the jump's descent, to avoid hyperextending your lower back and to prevent injury.

MOVE 18 | MOUNTAIN CLIMBING

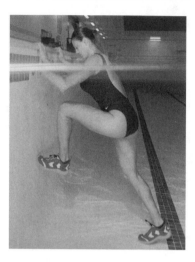

Starting Position: Move to the pool wall in chest-deep water, face the pool deck, and hold on to the edge with both hands.

Action:

1. Raise your left foot and put it on the wall of the pool at a comfortable height while keeping your right foot on the floor.

2. Jump up and switch the position of your legs.

3. Continue for 16 to 32 repetitions.

Safety Tips: Keep your knees slightly bent and your abdominals pulled in firmly. Avoid this exercise if you have neck pain.

SKI AND JACK COMBO

Starting Position: Stand in waist- to chest-deep water. Start with your right foot out in front of your body and your left foot back; reach your left arm out in front (but under the water) and reach your right arm back (figure *a*).

Action:

1. Hop up and bring your right leg forward while you press your left leg all the way back. At the same time, scoop your left palm forward as you press your right palm back.

2. Hop up and switch legs and arms: Bring your left leg forward as you push your right leg back. At the same time, scoop your right palm forward and press your left palm back.

3. Jump up and land in a wide stance, with your knees bent and your heels on the pool floor with your right heel pressed out to the side. Your toes should be slightly pointed out to the sides. At the same time, press your palms out to either side. Keep your hands under the water (figure *b*).

4. Jump up and bring your feet together. Land with bent knees. At the same time, press your palms toward one another behind your buttocks.

5. Repeat the full sequence for 8 sets on both sides.

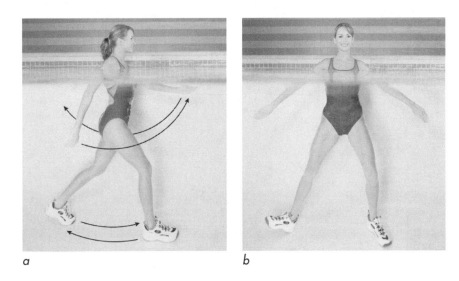

a   b

Safety Tips: Keep your abdominals and buttocks contracted to brace your spine in neutral alignment. Keep your chest lifted and your shoulder blades back and down.

Starting Position: Stand in water that reaches to your rib cage or chest. Begin in the neutral position, with your spine braced; keep your arms bent and your elbows at your sides. Imagine a ski slope with mogul humps.

Action:

1. Jump up, tucking your torso, lifting both knees, and squeezing the abdominals firmly while you press your palms to the right in order to jump left (figure a).
2. Bring your feet back down, pressing your heels to the floor and bending your knees.
3. Jump up, tucking your torso, lifting both knees, and squeezing the abdominals firmly while you press your palms to the left in order to jump right (figure b).
4. Bring your feet back down, pressing your heels to the floor and bending your knees.

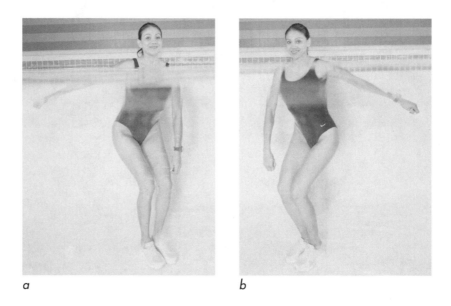

a   b

Variation: Once you have developed enough abdominal strength and corresponding level of fitness to perform the Mogul Hop without risking injury, start with 4 repetitions at moderate tempo (for example, to music with 130 beats per minute). For variety, jump forward 4 to 8 times and then backward 4 to 8 times.

Safety Tips: The jump requires a firm contraction of your abdominals and buttocks as well as a water power hop that incorporates the push-off training principle of plyometrics. Therefore, it should be performed once you have gained a basic level of fitness and can control the exercise. During these exercises, your abdominal muscles work together with your back, buttocks, and hips for coordinated strength. Keep your abdominals pulled in firmly, even during the jump's descent, to avoid hyperextending your lower back and to prevent injury.

KNEE-LIFT PRESS-BACK

Starting Position: Stand in waist- to chest-deep water, with your feet shoulder-width apart and your hands at your sides.

Action:
1. Press your palms back behind you as you lift your left knee toward your chest (figure *a*).
2. Bring your palms forward as you press your left leg back behind you (figure *b*). Repeat steps 1 and 2 four times; then bring your feet together.
3. Press your palms behind you and lift your knee toward your chest.
4. Bring both palms forward as you press your right leg behind you.
5. Repeat steps 3 and 4 four times.

Variation: Instead of bringing both arms forward, alternate arms as shown.

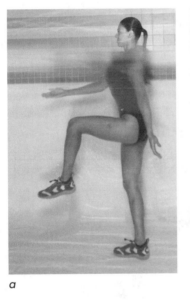
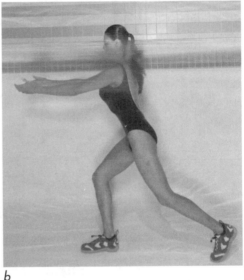

a   *b*

Safety Tips: As you lift your knee, avoid allowing your back to round or your hips and pelvis to dip under. As you press your leg back, keep your abdominals pulled in firmly to avoid hyperextending your lower back and to prevent injury.

ROCKING HORSE

Starting Position: Place your right foot in front of your left foot. Adopt the braced neutral position.

Action:

1. Standing on your left foot, lift your right knee toward your chest and press both palms down past your hips, keeping your arms relatively straight (figure *a*).
2. Hop forward onto your right leg as you kick your left heel up and behind you toward your buttocks. At the same time, swing both arms forward, with your palms facing up (figure *b*).
3. Repeat steps 1 and 2 for 8 sets.
4. Standing on your right foot, lift your left knee toward your chest and press both palms down past your hips.
5. Hop forward onto your left leg as you kick your right heel up and behind you toward your buttocks. At the same time, press both palms forward.
6. Repeat steps 3 and 4 for 8 sets.

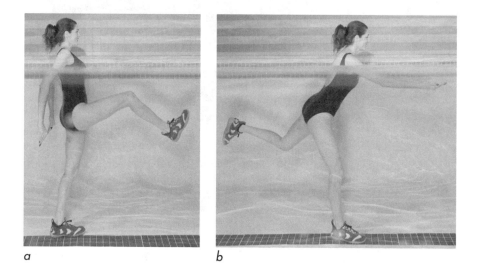

a   *b*

Safety Tips: In the Rocking Horse exercise, it is especially important to brace your spine to avoid arching your lower back. Hold your abdominals firmly in the tucked position and contract your buttocks. Keep your torso upright, your chest open, and your shoulder blades back and down; breathe deeply. Avoid arching your lower back, especially as you kick up your back heel, and do not lean forward and back.

LUNGE AND CENTER

Starting Position: Start with your hands at your sides and your body in the neutral position.

Action:

1. Jump up and turn your whole torso right as you swing both arms out to the right, palms first. At the same time, squeeze your abdominal muscles and thrust your left leg back (figure *a*).

2. Jump up, turn your torso back to the starting position, and bring both feet together at the center. Bring your arms to your sides (figure *b*).

3. Jump up and turn your whole torso to the left as you swing both arms out to the left, palms first. At the same time, thrust your right leg back (figure *c*).

4. Jump up, turn your torso back to the starting position, and bring both feet together at the center. Bring your arms to your sides.

5. Repeat 8 to 16 times.

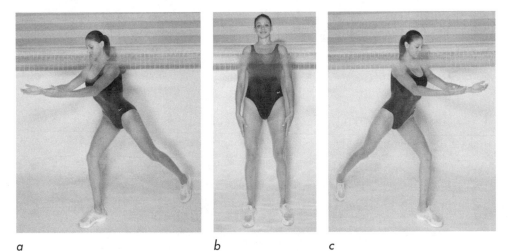

a   *b*   *c*

Variations:

- To reduce intensity, perform the movements without jumping; instead, pivot on your toes as you press your leg back and turn your whole torso. Step together to bring both feet back to the center.

- To increase intensity, do the following between lunges: Pull your abdominals in firmly, tuck your torso, and bring both knees toward your chest before bringing your feet together at the center. Or bound forward for 4 repetitions, then perform Lunge and Center once to each side, bound back for 4 repetitions, and perform Lunge and Center once to each side.

Safety Tips: Each time you thrust your leg back, tuck your abdominals in firmly to protect your spine. Focus on keeping your chest open and your shoulder blades back and down.

LUNGE KICK SQUARE

Starting Position: Start with your hands at your sides and your body in the neutral position.

Action:

1. Lunge right (figure *a*) and then left (figure *b*), as in Lunge and Center (Move #23). Propel yourself off the floor by adding a jump between. After the left lunge, remain facing to the left.
2. Kick your right leg forward (figure *c*) from the hip and then your left leg (figure *d*).
3. Repeat the sequence until you have lunged and kicked while facing in all four directions. Then repeat in the opposite direction, lunging left and then right.

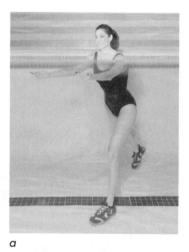

a

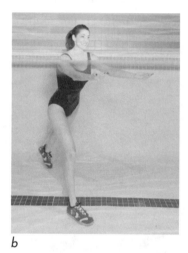

b

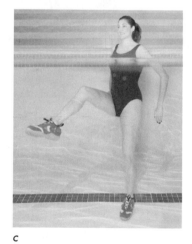

c

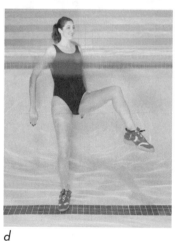

d

Safety Tips: Kick only as high as you can without your back rounding out, your hips and pelvis dipping forward, or your tailbone tucking under. If that is happening, keep your leg lower and your torso upright and contract your abdominals firmly. Each time you thrust your leg back for the lunge, tuck your abdominals in firmly to protect your spine. Focus on keeping your chest open and your shoulder blades back and down.

JUMP TWIST

Starting Position: Start in the neutral position with your elbows bent, your hands out in front, palms flat or cupped with thumbs up.

Action:

1. Tuck your torso, crouching slightly, and push off the bottom of the pool to jump up. While in the air, turn your whole body one-half turn to the right by pressing both hands to the left, keeping your elbows near your waist (figure *a*).
2. Coil again and push off the bottom of the pool while you press both hands to the right, keeping your elbows near your waist. At the same time, turn your body one-half turn to the left (figure *b*).
3. Repeat steps 1 and 2 eight times.

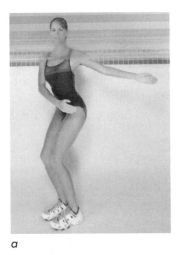 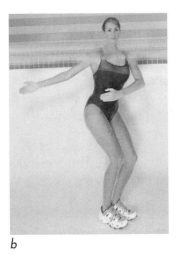

a   b

Variation: To increase intensity and reduce stress on your lower back, first bound forward for 4 repetitions and then perform the Jump Twist once in each direction; bound back for 4 repetitions and do the Jump Twist once in each direction. This allows you to realign your spine between Jump Twists.

Safety Tip: Keep your body stabilized and aligned in the neutral position. The arms propel the twisting motion and the torso and legs turn as a unit.

Flotation Aerobics

Flotation equipment helps your workout with the exercises that follow. Choose from this equipment: flotation belt, water exercise vest, noodle, or cuffs. Here are some helpful hints.

- Use your arms in opposition to your legs: When your right leg kicks forward, bring your left arm forward and vice versa.

- If you are using a flotation belt, tighten the belt snugly enough to keep it from riding up when you move to deep water but loosely enough to permit comfortable breathing. Wet vests are specially designed to prevent the flotation equipment from riding up and provide a greater sense of balance.

- Upper-arm flotation cuffs are inexpensive and they give you a greater sense of confidence if flotation belts make you feel unbalanced. If you have back pain, you may find these cuffs particularly comfortable. If you have neck pain, opt for a flotation belt or vest.

- Noodles are inexpensive, versatile, and fun to use.

MOVE 26 AQUA SKI

Equipment: Use a flotation belt, water exercise vest, or cuffs.

Starting Position: Move to water deep enough to bring your feet off the bottom of the pool. Squeeze your abdominal and buttocks muscles and press your feet down until your legs point straight downward. Bring your right leg forward and your left leg back. Press your left arm forward and your right arm back.

Action:

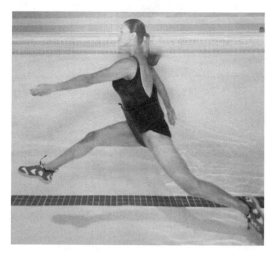

1. Using a gliding motion, simulate cross-country ski actions. Bring your right leg forward as you thrust your left leg behind you. Bring your left arm forward at the same time, and push your right arm back. Strive to reach a full range of motion that is controlled and comfortable; avoid using short, quick, choppy repetitions. Press your front leg all the way forward and your back leg all the way back.

2. Switch legs and arms with a gliding motion.

3. Repeat 8 to 16 times.

Variations:

- To reduce intensity, keep your knees bent.
- For higher intensity, propel your body across the pool. Use cupped palms to pull the water back, and slice your hand through the water when you bring your hand forward.

Safety Tips: Pull in your abdominals firmly and brace your spine with your buttocks muscles to protect your lower back. Keep your chest open and lifted and your shoulder blades back and down.

FLOATING SIDE SCISSORS

MOVE
27

Equipment: Use flotation belt, water exercise vest, or cuffs.

Starting Position: Move to water deep enough to bring your feet off the pool bottom. Squeeze your abdominal and buttocks muscles and press your feet down until your legs point straight downward (figure *a*).

Action:

1. Scissor your legs outward to a comfortable distance apart (figure *b*). Press your arms out to each side at the same time.
2. Bring your legs together and your hands to your sides.
3. Repeat 8 to 16 times.

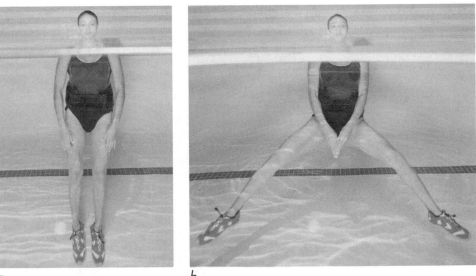

a *b*

Variation: Bend your knees slightly to increase the turbulence of the water and the intensity of the movement as you push and pull your legs through the water.

Safety Tips: Pull your abdominals firmly and brace your spine with your buttocks muscles to protect your lower back. Keep your chest lifted and your shoulder blades back and down.

BACK FLOAT KICK AND SQUIGGLE

Equipment: Use flotation belt, water exercise vest, or cuffs.

Starting Position: Move to water deep enough to bring your feet off the pool bottom. Lie back, with your spine braced in the neutral position between contracted abdominals and buttocks.

Action:

1. Flutter kick in a small motion from your hips and propel yourself the length of the pool. Keep your feet under the water.
2. Squiggle your arms in an "S"-like motion at your sides. Repeat as many times as enjoyable.

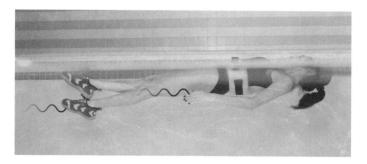

Variation: If you don't mind a wet head, you can simulate the backstroke to increase intensity.

Safety Tips: Look over your shoulder periodically to avoid collision with other swimmers. For neck support, add a flotation cervical collar.

VERTICAL FROG BOB

Equipment: Use flotation belt, noodle, water exercise vest, or cuffs.

Starting Position: Move to water deep enough to bring your feet off the pool bottom. Bring your feet down so that your legs point straight downward.

Action:

1. Firmly squeeze your abdominal and buttocks muscles and, from the hips, draw both knees powerfully toward your chest. Press your palms toward each other in front of you as you tuck (figure a).
2. Bring your feet wide apart while straightening your legs toward the pool bottom (figure b). Press your palms outward and then down to your sides as you bring your feet apart and straighten your legs.
3. Swiftly glide your legs together.
4. Repeat the sequence 8 times.

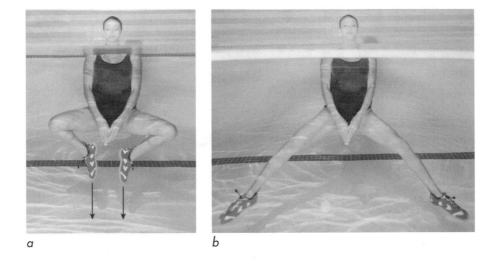

a   b

Variation: For increased intensity, perform the same exercise horizontally, on your back, while crossing the pool.

Safety Tip: Maintain control of your neck and torso stabilizer muscles to stay in neutral position throughout in order to make this move benefit, rather than strain, your back and neck.

VERTICAL FLUTTER KICK

MOVE
30

Equipment: Use flotation belt, noodle, water exercise vest, or cuffs.

Starting Position: Move to water deep enough to bring your feet off the pool bottom. Bring your feet down so that your legs point straight downward. Circle your hands around each other in front of your chest in a "mixing" motion.

Action:

1. Flutter kick your legs from the hips in a short, brisk motion.
2. Continue to flutter for as long as you can maintain your neutral stabilization. Gradually add more time as you become more proficient or intersperse 10 seconds of performing Vertical Flutter Kick throughout your flotation aerobics sequence.

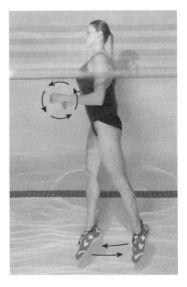

Variation: Vertical Flutter Spin: Rotate in a small circle as you flutter kick.

Safety Tip: Maintain your torso and neck stabilization in neutral position throughout. If you continue past the point of fatigue of your stabilizers, you may strain your back and neck.

FLOATING MOUNTAIN CLIMB

Equipment: Use flotation belt, noodle, water exercise vest, or cuffs.

Starting Position: Move to water deep enough to bring your feet off the pool bottom. Bring your feet down so that your legs point straight downward.

Action:

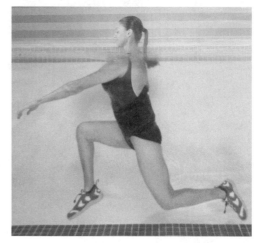

1. Bring your right knee forward and up. Extend your leg way out in front of you as if you were hiking up a steep incline. At the same time, press all the way back with your left leg. Simultaneously pump your arms, with your hands palms first against the water, in opposition to the movement of your legs.

2. Switch legs and repeat, alternating legs, and arms, while crossing the pool.

3. Work up to 16 repetitions.

Safety Tip: Maintain firmly contracted abdominal and buttocks muscles and somewhat vertical torso position to protect your lower back.

BICYCLE PUMP

Equipment: Use flotation belt, water exercise vest, noodle, or cuffs.

Starting Position: Move to water deep enough to bring your feet off the pool bottom. Bring your feet down so that your legs point straight downward. Position the body upright and vertical.

Action:

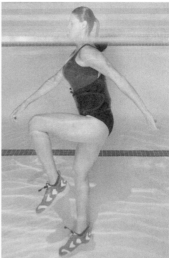

1. Contract your abdominal and buttocks muscles.

2. Draw one knee toward your chest, keeping your back flat and straight, while you extend the other leg toward the pool bottom.

3. Switch legs.

4. Repeat the sequence briskly 16 times.

Variation: To increase intensity, increase resistance of the surface area by flexing your foot, rather than pointing your toes, so that your ankle forms a right angle.

Safety Tip: Keep neutral posture, with your abdominal muscles contracted, your chest lifted and open, your shoulder blades back and down, and your back flat in order to protect your spine.

CAN-CAN SOCCER KICK

Equipment: Use flotation belt, noodle, water exercise vest, or cuffs.

Starting Position: Move to water deep enough to bring your feet off the pool bottom. Imagine that you are sitting in a chair; adopt that position. Space your knees about 6 inches (15 cm) apart and bend both legs to 90 degrees. Firmly contract your abdominal and buttocks muscles.

Action:

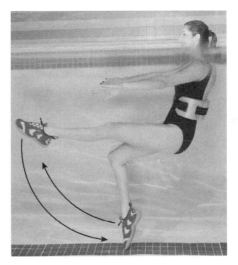

1. Keep your feet and knees under the water and your hips stationary. Instead of kicking from the hips, extend your leg from the knee, kicking your leg out straight.
2. Bend your right leg to 90 degrees. At the same time, kick out with your left leg.
3. Alternately kick and bend each leg for 16 repetitions.

Variations:

- To increase intensity by increasing the resistance of the surface area, point your toes.
- For reduced intensity, flex your ankle.

Safety Tip: Avoid hyperextending at the knee: Stop the kick at the point where your leg is straight and before your knee starts to bend the other way.

Advanced Conditioning Techniques

Use the advanced variations to increase the challenge as you become more fit. See chapter 7, Intensifying Workouts, if you are interested in sampling the excitement of powerful peak aerobic plyometrics for cardiovascular fitness and neuromuscular power. Add advanced, explosive moves, such as Plyometrics Jacks and Dolphin Jump, when you are ready to obtain a higher level of fitness. Plyometrics employ powerful push-offs from the pool floor to raise your cardiorespiratory intensity and build balance and coordination skills.

Aerobic Cool-Down

Use the same exercises as those described under Warm-Up Aerobics at the beginning of this chapter. Progressively shorten the range of motion, reduce traveling, and minimize jumping as you gradually lower the intensity of your aerobic moves. Cool-down is an essential component of the aerobic exercise sequence that allows your body to adapt gradually to the decrease in cardio-respiratory demand. Skipping the cool-down can increase the chance of the cardiovascular events or injuries at any age. Finish every water exercise session with a final cool-down stretch sequence, as described in chapter 4, Warming Up and Cooling Down. Without the final cool-down stretches, your risk of soreness or injury increases significantly.

CHAPTER 6

Strengthening and Toning

Muscle strengthening and toning are important for more than aesthetic reasons. Studies show that regular, consistent fitness activities to improve and maintain muscular strength can prevent injuries and increase your chance of maintaining physical independence and mobility as you age. Exercises that incorporate higher resistance for fewer repetitions increase strength and also produce muscular endurance benefits. More repetitions at lower resistance primarily improve muscular endurance, meaning the number of repetitions that can be completed before the muscle fatigues.

Muscle strengthening and toning exercises also increase total lean body mass and improve the ratio of lean to fatty tissue. Therefore, as you develop a greater percentage of muscle tissue, your body metabolizes more calories at rest and while you are exercising. For that reason, muscle strengthening and toning are an important component of any weight management plan. Research has shown that people who engage in muscle strengthening and toning activities two or three times a week are more successful in losing weight and keeping it off over the long term than those who don't.

Muscle training in water increases muscle strength, endurance, and tone. If you want to emphasize muscular strength over endurance, after you have mastered the basics, add resistance equipment, as described in chapter 2, Preparing for Water Workouts. Focus your attention on positioning your body and exerting with the muscles identified for each exercise. Each exercise instruction specifies the muscle group used and explains equipment options, body position, muscle action, proper breathing, and variations. Ideally, you should perform strengthening and toning exercises every other day. Skip a day in between strengthening workouts to allow for rest and recovery of the muscles worked. This time is needed for your body to complete the processes necessary to build firmer, stronger, more capable muscle and tendon tissue. If you perform resistance or strengthening exercises with the same muscle group two days in a row, you are not allowing enough time for the body's adaptation process and injury is likely to occur. Familiarize yourself with the following definitions of fitness training before you begin.

Contract—Squeeze, firm, or tighten the muscle you are working to mobilize the muscle fibers into action.

Isolate—Focus your energy on the muscle you are working and minimize motion in the rest of your body.

Flex—Decrease the angle between two ends of a joint, for example, by bending your knee.

Extend—Increase the angle of the joint, for example, by straightening your elbow.

Abduct—Move a limb away from the midline of your body.

Adduct—Move a limb toward the midline of your body.

Core Strength—Core strength is the *balanced* development of the muscles that stabilize and move your torso, including your abdominals and muscles of your back. The goal is to develop the deep internal muscles of your torso so that all of the muscles are moving in the most efficient relation to each other. Development of core strength requires training the abdominal, pelvic, buttocks, neck, and back muscles that surround the core area of your body so that all of the torso joints, including the spine, are surrounded by a firm and powerful support structure of muscle bundles running in different directions. The core muscles act as shock absorbers for jumps, rebounds, or plyometric exercises; they stabilize your body and represent a link, or transmitter, between your legs and arms.

Lower Body

Lower-body exercises tone and strengthen your hips, thighs, buttocks, and lower legs (review the muscle diagrams in figure 3.6 on page 51), producing a sleeker body appearance and, when performed properly, helping prevent knee and back pain. Concentrate on learning proper body position to enhance your results and prevent painful injuries associated with poor technique. If you focus on contracting the muscles indicated in the "muscle focus" for each exercise, you can achieve improvements more readily.

Advanced Conditioning Techniques

After you have mastered the lower-body conditioning exercises in this chapter, you can add more sets of repetitions to increase your workout. Add power to your advanced workout. See Powering Your Way to Fitness, beginning on page 130 in chapter 7, Intensifying Workouts, for excellent Power Moves for advanced lower-body toning—such as the Squat Step and the Squat Knee Lift. You can employ Power Moves after your aerobic exercise to tone up and cool down while keeping your heart rate in the low end of your aerobic target zone.

OUTER- AND INNER-THIGH SCISSORS

Equipment: If your torso and lower-body muscles are basically strong, you may wish to wear resistance cuffs, fins, or boots on your lower legs or feet to increase intensity.

Muscle Focus: This move exercises the muscles of your hip and your inner and outer thighs.

Starting Position: Perform this exercise in waist- to chest-deep water. Stand with your side to the wall, and hold on to the pool deck with one hand for balance. Perform one set with your toes pointing straight ahead and one set with your toes pointing out. Keep both hip bones pointing straight ahead, at equal height from the floor. Be sure to contract your abdominal muscles throughout the movement in order to maintain this position. Adopt the braced neutral position.

Action:

1. Perform hip abduction: Lift your outside leg out to the side. Do not lean toward or away from the pool wall (figure *a*).
2. Perform hip adduction: Contract the muscles of your inner thigh to bring your feet back together (figure *b*).
3. Repeat 8 to 16 times.
4. Change sides and repeat the exercise the same number of times with the other leg.

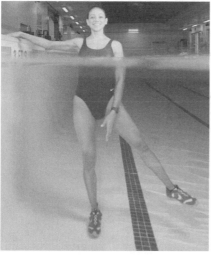

a

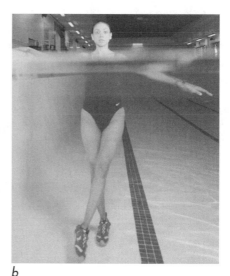

b

Variations:

- Scoop your outside palm in toward your body as you kick out. Then scoop your palm out to the side as you bring your leg back down to the starting position.
- If you have strong, stable torso muscles and no lower-back pain, vary your strength work by crossing your leg in front of your stationary foot 4 times and in back of your foot 4 times.

(continued)

Safety Tips: Keep your chest lifted, your shoulder blades back and down, and your torso straight up and evenly balanced front to back and left to right. Lift only as high as you can without leaning to one side or moving your torso. Lift your leg only and avoid elevating your hip. Put your hand on your outside hip to help keep the hip stable. No motion should occur at your waist or neck. Contract your abdominal and buttocks muscles to protect your lower back. If you experience back pain, keep your leg lower on each lift.

<table>
<tr><td>MOVE
35</td><td></td></tr>
</table>

MOVE 35 — FORWARD-AND-BACK LEG GLIDE

Equipment: If your torso and lower-body muscles are strong, you may wish to wear cuffs, fins, or boots on your lower legs or feet to increase intensity.

Muscle Focus: This move exercises the muscles of your hip, buttocks, and the front and back of your thighs.

Starting Position: Perform this exercise in waist- to chest-deep water. Stand with your side to the wall, and hold on to the pool deck with one hand to aid your balance. Contract your abdominal and buttocks muscles to brace yourself in the neutral position.

Action:

1. Flex at the hip: Lift your inside leg forward from the hip to a comfortable height (figure a).
2. Extend at the hip: Reverse the direction of movement and press your leg backward only as far as you can without arching your lower back. Place your hand on your lower back to monitor your position (figure b).
3. Repeat the sequence 8 to 16 times. Turn around and repeat steps 1 and 2 with the other leg for the same number of repetitions.

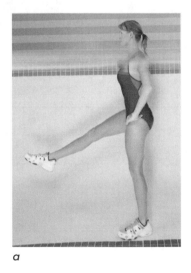
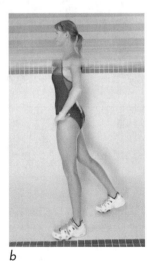

a   b

Variations:

- Bend your knee or slow down the movement if you wish to decrease the intensity of this exercise.
- To add upper-body activity, scoop your palm backward as you kick forward and scoop forward as you press your leg back.

Safety Tips: Contract your abdominal muscles firmly as you press your leg back. Keep your chest lifted, your shoulder blades down and back, and your torso up straight. Limit the height of the backward kick to the point where you can maintain the position without arching your back: Higher is not better. No motion should occur at your torso, waist, or neck.

KNEE KICK

Equipment: If your torso and lower-body muscles are strong, you may wish to wear resistance cuffs, fins, or boots on your lower legs or feet to increase intensity.

Muscle Focus: This move exercises the front and back of your thighs.

Starting Position: Perform this exercise in waist- to chest-deep water. Stand with your side to the wall, and hold on to the pool deck with one hand for balance. Contract your abdominal and buttock muscles to brace yourself in the neutral position. Keep your chest lifted and your shoulder blades back and down. Raise your leg to a right angle at the hip and knee.

Action:

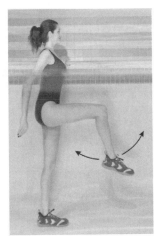

1. Contract the front of your thigh and kick your leg toward the surface of the pool while pushing against the resistance of the water.
2. Contract the back of your thigh and squeeze your buttocks as you flex (bend) at the knee.
3. Repeat 8 to 16 times. Turn around and repeat the same number of times with the other leg.

Variations:

- If you find it hard to hold your leg up, use the outside leg, reach behind your thigh, and support your leg as you kick. Be sure to stand straight, with your abdominals contracted, your chest lifted, and your shoulder blades back and down.
- Increase intensity by pointing the toes of your kicking leg. Reduce intensity by kicking with your foot flexed (hold your ankle at a right angle).

Safety Tips: Avoid locking your knee when you straighten your leg. Eliminate this exercise if you have knee pain; add it to your routine when your knee is healed and free of pain.

RUNNER'S STRIDE

Equipment: If your torso and lower-body muscles are strong and you suffer no knee pain, you may wish to add resistance cuffs, fins, or boots to your lower legs or feet to increase intensity.

Muscle Focus: This move exercises your hip, buttocks, and the front and back of your thigh.

Starting Position: Perform this exercise in waist- to chest-deep water. Stand with your side to the wall, and hold on to the pool deck with one hand for balance. Contract your abdominal and buttocks muscles to brace your spine in the neutral position.

Action:

1. Lift your leg to a right angle at the hip and knee (figure *a*).
2. Kick your foot toward the surface (figure *b*).
3. Press your straight leg down and back behind you.
4. Kick your heel toward your buttocks.
5. Raise your leg to a right angle at the hip and knee.
6. Repeat the full sequence 8 to 16 times. Turn around and repeat the same number of times with the other leg.

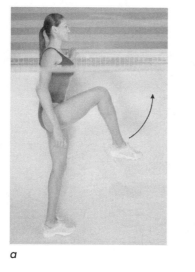
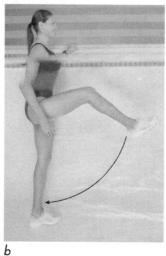

a   b

Safety Tips: Focus on maintaining a firmly supported neutral position without leaning forward or back or arching your lower back. Avoid hyperextending (over-straightening) your knee. Eliminate this exercise if you tend to experience knee pain; add it to your routine when your knee is fully healed and free of pain.

Equipment: If your torso and lower-body muscles are strong and you suffer no hip pain, you may wish to wear resistance cuffs, fins, or boots on your lower legs or feet to increase intensity.

Muscle Focus: This move exercises your hip and buttocks.

Starting Position: Perform this exercise in waist- to chest-deep water. Stand with your side to the wall, and hold onto the pool deck with one hand for balance. Contract your abdominal and buttocks muscles to brace your spine in the neutral position. Raise your outside knee in front to form a right angle at the hip and knee.

Action:

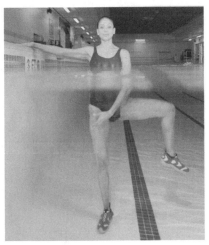

1. Press your knee out to the side.
2. Press your knee back to the standing position.
3. Repeat 8 to 16 times. Turn around and repeat the same number of times with the other leg.

Variation: This move helps improve lower-body alignment because you perform a smooth motion: Lift your knee, press it out toward the wall, bring it back to the starting position, and put your foot down. Repeat the exercise 8 to 16 times on each side.

Safety Tips: Protect your hip and back by moving slowly and with control. Avoid turning your torso: Place your hand on your abdomen to make sure that you are not twisting your torso as you press your knee out and in. To protect your knee joint, avoid bending your knee beyond 90 degrees of flexion.

PIVOTED DIP

Muscle Focus: This move exercises your buttocks and the front and back of your thighs.

Standing Position: Perform this exercise in waist-deep water. Stand with your side to the wall, and hold on to the pool deck with one hand for balance. Squeeze your abdominals and buttocks to brace your spine in the neutral position. Place one leg behind the other and reach forward with your outside arm, with your palm facing forward.

Action:

1. Lower your back knee toward the pool floor as you press your outside palm down past your side (figure *a*).

2. Press yourself back up, using the muscles of the front leg as you press your arm forward, with your palm up (figure *b*).

3. Repeat 8 times, pivot turn on your toes to switch sides, and repeat 8 more times. Add more repetitions and sets of repetitions gradually as you become stronger.

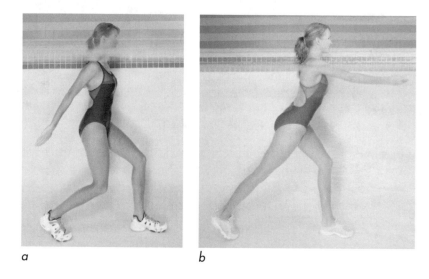

a　　　　　　　　　　　*b*

Variation: Start by performing this exercise with your hand on your hip to avoid confusion that can accompany trying to coordinate your arms and legs. Later, add the arm movements to help build coordination.

Safety Tip: Be sure that your front knee is positioned over your heel, not pushed forward over your toes.

WALL SQUAT

Muscle Focus: This move exercises your hips, buttocks, and the front and back of your thighs. It helps build strong knee stability.

Starting Position: Perform this exercise in waist-deep water. Stand facing the wall or ladder, and hold on with both hands. Bring your feet shoulder-width apart or hip-width apart, with your knees pointing the same direction as your first and second toes. Your toes should be pointing straight ahead or turned out slightly. Contract your abdominal and buttocks muscles to brace your spine in the neutral position.

Action:

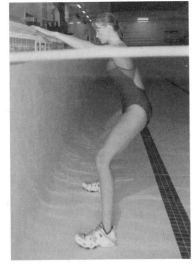

1. Lift your chest and push your buttocks back and down, as if you are lowering yourself toward a chair placed 1 foot (30 cm) or so behind you. Squat to about one-third of the way toward the imaginary chair.

2. Slowly press through your feet, using your buttocks and thigh muscles, and come back to a standing upright position.

3. Perform 8 to 16 repetitions.

Variation: Bring your feet farther apart and turn them out slightly. Complete 8 to 10 repetitions.

Safety Tips: Contract your abdominal muscles firmly and avoid arching your back. Keep your knees back behind your toes as you squat. Squat less deeply if you have difficulty keeping your knees behind your toes.

Muscle Focus: This move exercises your hips, buttocks, and the front and back of your thighs. It helps build strong knee stability.

Starting Position: Perform this exercise in waist-deep water. Stand facing the wall or ladder, and hold on with both hands. Bring your feet shoulder-width apart or wider, with your knees pointing the same direction as your first and second toes. Your toes should be pointing straight ahead or turned out slightly. Contract your abdominal and buttocks muscles to brace your spine in the neutral position (figure a).

Action:

1. Perform a Wall Squat.
2. Slowly press through your feet, using your buttocks and thigh muscles. As you press yourself back up, abduct at the thigh and touch your left toe out to the left side while keeping your leg straight (figure b).
3. Bring your leg back as you squat again and repeat steps 1 and 2, but lift and touch out with the right leg.
4. Perform 8 to 16 repetitions.

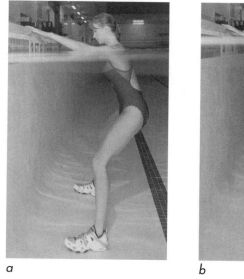
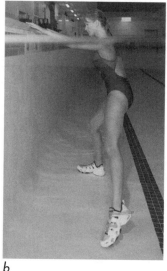

a   b

Variation: Bring your feet farther apart and turn them out slightly. Complete 8 to 10 repetitions.

Safety Tips: Contract your abdominal muscles firmly and avoid arching your back.

CALF LIFT

Muscle Focus: This move exercises the back of your calf and strengthens your feet.

Starting Position: Perform this exercise in waist- to chest-deep water. Face the pool deck, and hold on to the edge. Stand up straight an arm's length from the pool wall, with your feet shoulder-width apart and your knees relaxed. Contract your abdominal and buttocks muscles to brace your spine in the neutral position.

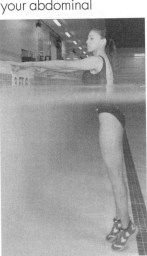

Action:

1. Raise yourself up onto your toes.
2. Slowly lower your heels to the floor.
3. Repeat 8 to 16 times.

Variations:

- Bring your feet farther apart and turn them out slightly. Complete 8 to 10 repetitions.
- Raise one knee and perform 8 to 10 repetitions on one leg and then repeat on the other.

Safety Tips: If your feel wobbly when you try the Calf Lift, perform this exercise by lifting one leg and pointing and flexing the lifted foot and then change legs and repeat. Include ankle rolls, and spell out the alphabet with your toes to improve flexibility and strength around the joints of your ankles and feet. You can hold on with one hand behind your lifted knee; be sure to brace yourself in neutral position and hold on to the pool wall.

TOE LIFT

Muscle Focus: This move exercises your shins.

Starting Position: Perform this exercise in waist- to chest-deep water. Face the pool deck, and hold on the edge. Stand up straight an arm's length from the pool wall, with your feet wider than shoulder-width apart and your knees flexed and relaxed. Squeeze your abdominal and buttocks muscles to brace your spine in neutral position. Point your feet out slightly to the sides.

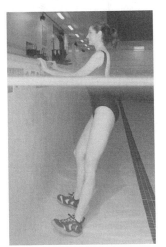

Action:

1. Lift your toes so that your forefoot lifts up, keeping your heels on the floor.
2. Press your toes back toward the floor.
3. Repeat 16 times.

Variation: Lift one foot at a time, tapping twice on one side and twice on the other. Repeat 8 times.

Safety Tip: Move slowly, smoothly, and deliberately, and make the muscles on the front of your leg do the work.

Upper Body

Good upper-body strength makes performing daily tasks easier and helps prevent injuries. The upper-body exercises work your chest, back, shoulders, and upper arms. Review figure 3.4 on page 50 to familiarize yourself with the location of the muscles used. Perform these exercises without equipment at first. Then, if you have no upper-body joint pains, add webbed gloves, disks, kickboards, or water bells for added strength and toning. Establish a solid level of strength before adding new resistance to your routine; to do otherwise may cause injury.

MOVE 44   CHEST AND UPPER-BACK GLIDE

Equipment: Use webbed gloves, water exercise bells, plastic plates, Frisbees, or paddles.

Muscle Focus: This move exercises your chest and upper body.

Starting Position: Perform this exercise in chest- to shoulder-deep water. Stand with one foot in front of the other at a comfortable distance apart that provides good stability. Contract your abdominal and buttocks muscles to brace your spine in neutral position. Keep your chest lifted and your shoulder blades down and back. Make a particular effort to keep your shoulder blades squeezed together and down. Your shoulders should be partly submerged.

Action:

1. Extend both arms out to the sides, with your palms facing forward (figure *a*).
2. Press both palms in toward one another, out in front of your chest (figure *b*).

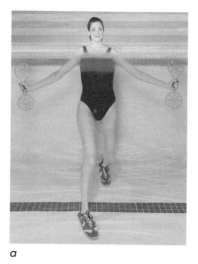
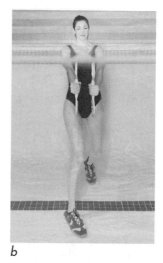

a   *b*

3. Turn your palms around and press back until your hands are even with your back.

4. Repeat the sequence for 8 to 16 repetitions.

Safety Tip: For greater stability, perform using one arm at a time, holding on to the pool edge, with your side toward the wall.

SPORT TRAINING RACKET SWEEP

Equipment: Use an old tennis racket or other sports equipment such as a lacrosse stick, Ping-Pong paddle, squash or racquet ball racquet. Be careful to avoid damaging the pool lining with the equipment.

Muscle Focus: This move conditions and trains the muscles used for your sport.

Starting Position: Perform this exercise in chest- to shoulder-deep water or water deep enough to submerge your equipment. Stand in a well-supported stance typically used in your sport. Contract your abdominals and buttocks to brace your spine in the neutral position. Keep your chest lifted and your shoulder blades down and back.

Action:

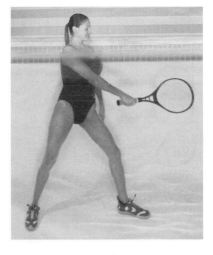

1. Perform a full swing or wrist flick, as used in your sport. Slow the speed down considerably to allow for the added resistance created by the viscosity of the water.

2. Change position often to simulate the stances and moves used in the sport and repeat the swings or wrist flicks in multiple directions.

Variation: To strengthen your rotator cuff at the shoulder, bend your elbow and keep your upper arm "pasted" down your side throughout the movement. Swing the racket frontward and backward *slowly*, as if the racket is a swinging door and your elbow and upper arm are the hinge. Swing slowly through your full, comfortable range of motion that does not lift your elbow away from your side or take your shoulder out of its "back and down" alignment. Work hard to keep your shoulder blades down and your abdominals firmly contracted.

Safety Tips: Be sure to slow down the speed considerably compared to doing the motion on land. It may seem as though you could move faster; however, you could be causing microtraumas if you are pushing too hard. Proper stabilization at your shoulder (and at your wrist for the tennis swing) prevents injury and strengthens your swing.

CHEST AND BACK PRESS

Equipment: Use noodle, webbed gloves, paddles, a small kickboard, water exercise bells, ball, plastic plates, or Frisbee.

Muscle Focus: This move exercises your chest and your midback and upper back.

Starting Position: Perform this exercise in chest- to shoulder-deep water. Stand with one foot in front of the other at a comfortable and stable distance apart. Contract your abdominals and buttocks to brace yourself in the neutral position. Keep your chest lifted and your shoulder blades down and back. Your shoulders should be partly submerged (figure *a*).

Action:

1. Contract the muscles of your shoulder blades to bring them together and down, and keep them in that position during the entire exercise (figure *b*). Press the equipment or your hands out in front of your chest, under the water.

2. Pull the disk, board, or your hands back toward your rib cage, and bring your elbows along your sides to a comfortable point behind your waist. Use the muscles of your midback.

3. Repeat 8 to 16 times.

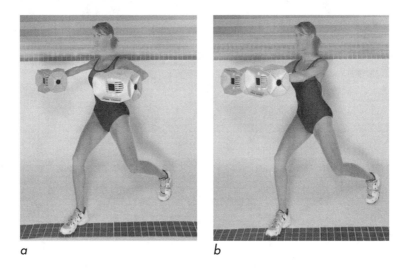

a   *b*

Variation: Perform the Chest and Back Press with your elbows elevated out to your sides.

Safety Tips: When you straighten your arms, keep a slight bend at your elbow to protect the elbow joint. Contract your abdominals firmly to stabilize your torso. For greater stability, perform the move with one arm at a time while you are holding on to the pool edge, with your side toward the wall.

DIAGONAL FRONT SHOULDER PRESS

Equipment: Use webbed gloves, water exercise bells, or paddles.

Muscle Focus: This move exercises the muscles of the shoulder's rotator cuff.

Starting Position: Perform this exercise in shoulder-deep water. Stand with your side next to the wall, and hold on to the pool edge with your hand for stability. Place your right (inside) foot back and your left (outside) foot forward at a comfortable distance apart. Contract your abdominal and buttocks muscles to brace your spine in the neutral position. Keep your chest lifted and your shoulder blades back and down. Your shoulders should be partly submerged. Reach out in front of your left leg with your left hand, and turn your palm down.

Action:

1. Press your left palm down and across your body toward your right thigh.
2. Lift your arm up toward the pool surface to return to the starting position.
3. Repeat 8 times. Then switch your position with a pivot turn and repeat 8 times.

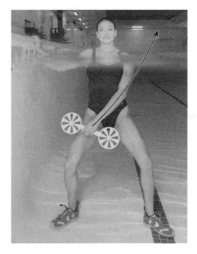

Safety Tip: Be sure to keep your wrist straight, in neutral alignment.

PIVOTED SHOULDER PRESS

Equipment: Use webbed gloves, water exercise bells, paddles, plastic plates, or Frisbees.

Muscle Focus: This move exercises the front and back of your shoulder.

Starting Position: Perform this exercise in chest- to shoulder-deep water. Stand with one foot in front of the other at a comfortable and stable distance apart. Contract your abdominal and buttocks muscles to brace your spine in the neutral position and stabilize your torso. Keep your chest lifted and your shoulder blades down and back. Bring both arms behind you, and turn your palms forward. Your shoulders should be partly submerged.

Action:

1. Press both palms forward toward the pool surface, out in front of your chest. Stop before you reach the surface of the water (figure a).
2. Turn your hands around and press your palms down past your sides behind your hips (figure b).
3. Repeat 8 to 16 times.

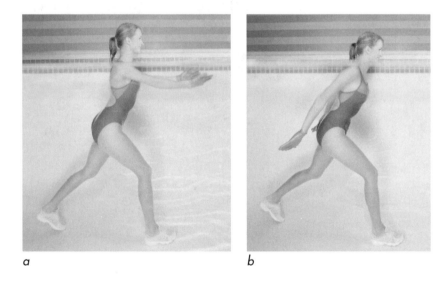

a   b

Safety Tips: Keep your shoulders down and back; as you press back, stop at the point of comfortable resistance. If your shoulders are coming up, you may be pressing too far back. Keep your hands under water during the entire exercise. For greater stability, perform the move with one arm at a time while you are holding on to the pool edge, with your side toward the wall.

SIDE ARM PUMP

Equipment: Use webbed gloves, water exercise bells, or paddles.

Muscle Focus: This move exercises the top and outside of your shoulder and the side of your torso, under your arms.

Starting Position: Perform this exercise in chest- to shoulder-deep water. Stand with one foot in front of the other at a comfortable and stable distance apart. Keep your arms at your sides, and contract your abdominal and buttocks muscles to brace your spine in the neutral position and stabilize your torso. Keep your chest lifted and your shoulder blades down and back.

Action:

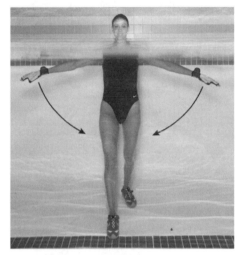

1. Slowly lift both arms out to your sides, with your palms up, toward the surface of the water.
2. Slowly press both arms down to your sides, with your palms down.
3. Repeat 8 to 16 times.

Variation: Lift both arms out to your sides and press them down behind your buttocks instead of pressing them down to your sides. Imagine that you are squeezing a beach ball behind your back.

Safety Tips: Keep your hands underwater throughout the entire exercise. For greater stability, perform the move with one arm at a time while you are holding on to the pool edge, with your side toward the pool wall. If you have neck pain, minimize this exercise by reducing speed and repetitions.

Equipment: Use webbed gloves, water exercise bells, paddles, plastic plates, or Frisbees.

Muscle Focus: This move exercises the front and back of your upper arms.

Starting Position: Perform this exercise in upper chest- to shoulder-deep water. Stand with one foot in front of the other at a comfortable and stable distance apart. Contract your abdominal and buttocks muscles to brace your spine in the neutral position and stabilize your torso. Keep your chest lifted and your shoulder blades down and back. Bring both arms behind you, and turn your palms to face forward. Keep your elbows behind your waist for this exercise.

Action:

1. Bend your elbows (figure *a*). Keeping your upper arms motionless, press your palms upward toward your shoulders in an arc. Avoid lifting your hands out of the water.

2. Turn your palms toward the pool bottom, and press down and back (figure *b*).

3. Repeat 8 to 16 times.

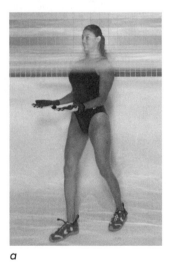 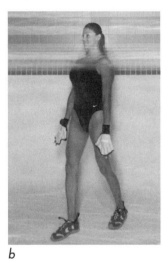

a   *b*

Safety Tips: Keep a slight bend in your elbow when you extend in order to protect your elbow joint. If you are using water exercise bells or paddles, you don't need to turn your hand around between steps 1 and 2. For greater stability, perform the move at poolside, using one arm at a time while you are holding on to the pool edge.

Abs

The exercises that follow enable you to employ the resistive qualities of water to create a healthier body core through stronger abdominal muscles that do a better job in stabilizing your body core. Use the mental images described here to improve muscle and movement control, positioning, and breathing during this stimulating progression of highly effective abdominal exercises. Before you begin, familiarize yourself with the actual muscles you are working (refer to figure 3.2 on page 48 in chapter 3) and focus your exertion on using those muscles during each exercise. Then review the "Exercise Precautions" on page 48.

Before you begin each abdominal exercise sequence, use this body awareness preparation to help you develop stronger abdominal control: Place your palms over the bottom half of both sides of your rib cage and contract the muscles over your rib cage. Use the imagery of closing an accordion or a fireplace bellows. Inhale and imagine that you can fill your abdominal cavity with air. Then contract your abdominals—the muscles above and below your navel and over your rib cage from your breastbone to your pelvis—and press your navel toward your spine as you exhale. At the same time, contract your buttocks somewhat to brace your spine in the neutral position. Place your hands over your abdomen to feel the muscles contract.

WALL-SIT CRUNCH AND ROCK-BELLY CRUNCH

Equipment: After you have mastered the basic exercise without equipment, add the use of buoyancy resistance by hugging a flotation belt, exercise ball, long barbell, kickboard, water ball, or pair of gallon jugs to your chest to increase resistance. The flotation exercise ball works best. Keep your shoulder blades down and back.

Starting Position: Move to chest-deep water and put your back to the pool wall. Slide a few inches down into a semiseated position and adopt the neutral position: Place your feet shoulder-width apart, with your knees bent, your abdominals firm, your chest lifted, and your shoulders back. Make sure that your knees are directly over your heels and that your knees are bent at 90 degrees or greater (figure a). You may need to move your feet to a position a bit farther from or closer to the pool wall.

Action:

1. Identify the upper and lower ends of the rectus abdominus muscle—at your breastbone and just above your pelvis. Become aware of the muscles that surround your rib cage, the external and internal obliques.

2. Shorten this distance between the two ends of your abdominals—your breastbone and your pelvis—as though you were closing an accordion. Contract the muscles over your rib cage while you compress your abdominals and obliques toward the midline at your navel (figure b). Strive to create a "rock belly" contraction by bringing the bottom of your rib cage closer to your hip bones as you "close the accordion."

3. Release the contraction slowly. Between repetitions, maintain a slight contraction in order to protect your back, by keeping your pelvis in a braced neutral position, and to work your abdominal muscle group more effectively.

4. Exhale on the contraction (close the accordion); inhale on the release. Refocus your attention on contracting your abdominal muscles while you execute proper breathing.

5. Repeat the sequence 8 to 32 times.

Variation: Advanced fitness enthusiasts are delighted with the results of performing the Wall-Sit Crunch with flotation equipment for resistance; it is a sequence that uses the buoyancy of water to duplicate the effects of weight training. Once your abdominal muscles are strong, challenge your torso by performing the exercise standing at midpool, away from the wall, using buoyant resistance equipment. You can reproduce the resistive qualities of a weight training machine by pressing against the flotation resistance of the buoys while contracting your abdominals.

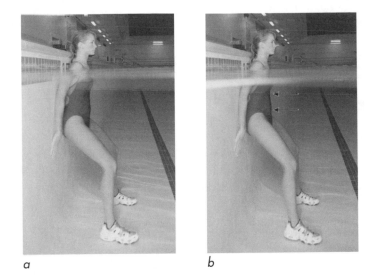

a   b

Hug the buoyancy equipment to your body, with your palms open and your fingers over the top. Walk to a depth where the equipment is slightly submerged. Continue with the abdominal crunch sequence and note the increased muscle energy required to partially submerge the equipment using the strength of the abdominals. Move the equipment to the left side of your rib cage and contract the muscles around the left side of your rib cage, the obliques. Repeat on the right side. Increase the number of repetitions as you become more proficient. For variety, use a count of 4 to move the body through abdominal contractions at four ranges of motion (imagine an elevator stopping at four floors), or hold contractions for 4 seconds and release.

If you use the reversed flotation belt, put both hands on top of the belt and perform the abdominal crunch. To focus on the muscles over your rib cage, put your left hand on the middle of your left thigh, with your right hand on the top of the belt. Squeeze your abdominal muscles to bring your torso slightly forward and to the right. Continue for several repetitions. Repeat the squeeze to the left.

Safety Tips: Avoid arching or hyperextending the lumbar spine during the release of the contraction. Check your alignment to be sure that the position of your pelvis is appropriate. Your pelvis should be in a neutral position, not tipped forward or backward, and braced firmly between an abdominal and buttocks contraction. Avoid moving up and down in a sitting motion, which can defeat the purpose of the exercise. Give yourself a few weeks or months to master each progressively more challenging stage of this exercise.

Equipment: A flotation belt or cuffs, or even a pair of plastic gallon jugs, can enhance this exercise for beginning, intermediate, and advanced exercisers.

Starting Position: Stand with your back to the pool wall, outstretch your arms, and place your palms on the wall behind you or put on the flotation belt or cuffs. Lie back, extending your body so that you are floating face up on your back. Extend your legs out in front of you just below the surface of the water (figure a). Keep your knees slightly bent and avoid bringing your knees toward your chest: The action is all in the shortening of your abdominal muscles; not much movement occurs.

Action:

1. Contract your abdominals while you are exhaling. Using your abdominal muscles, shorten the distance between your breastbone and pelvis; think about pressing your navel toward your backbone (figure b). If this is the first time you have performed this kind of exercise, you may not notice any movement at all until your muscles get stronger.

2. Extend your body. Avoid arching your back each time that you extend your body to a straightened position.

3. Exhale as you contract your abdominal muscles and then inhale as you release them.

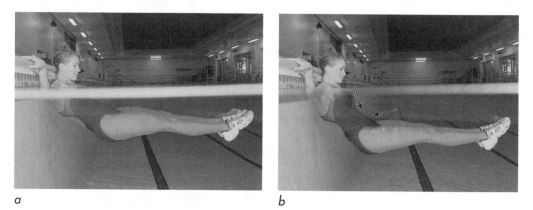

a   b

Variation: Place a long-handled flotation barbell beneath your knees or ankles to add greater challenge to the flotation curl or to assist you in keeping your legs floating if they tend to sink.

The Oblique Floating Curl helps work the external and internal oblique muscles (the muscles on your sides and rib cage) and increases the water resistance against your abdominal muscles. Here's how to do it:

1. Place the sole of your left foot against your right thigh or shin. Bend your right leg.

2. Contract the muscles of your abdomen to bring the left side of your rib cage and your breastbone closer to your left hip bone. Avoid rolling your shoulder forward; keep your shoulder blades down and back.

3. Repeat the move 4 to 8 times and then switch the position to work the opposite side for 4 to 8 repetitions. Over time, when your torso muscles feel stronger, gradually add more repetitions: Intersperse 2 or 3 sets of 8 repetitions throughout your abdominal workout.

For a more challenging and torso-strengthening variation of the Oblique Floating Curl, use two long-handled flotation barbells. Float on your back, extend your arms overhead with both hands clasped on the barbell, and place your ankles on a second barbell, about shoulder-width apart. Slowly contract the muscles of your sides to form a sideways jackknife with your body by squeezing the muscles on your left side; slowly return your body to a straight line position. Keep your abdominal muscles firmly contracted throughout the exercise. Perform 4 to 8 repetitions and then repeat on the other side. The Oblique Floating Curl challenges your torso and creates a stronger core that is more resilient to back pain and injuries.

Safety Tip: Focus on the muscle energy of shortening the distance between your breastbone and pelvis while you are contracting your abdominals to isolate the abdominal muscles.

SITTING V

MOVE
53

Equipment: A flotation belt, cuffs, or empty plastic gallon jugs can enhance this experience for beginning, intermediate, and advanced exercisers.

Starting Position: While holding on to the pool wall or using a flotation device, lie back, extending your body so that you are floating faceup on your back.

Action:

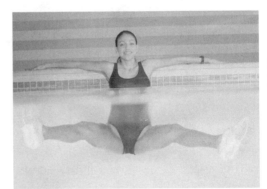

1. Bring your legs out to the sides (open the V). At the same time, contract (squeeze) your abdominal muscles to bring your torso into a partially seated position, with your legs extended to either side.

2. Lie back, bring your legs together, and relax your abdominals.

3. Perform 8 to 16 repetitions.

Proper Breathing: Exhale as you contract your abdominal muscles and inhale as you release them.

Variation: As you get stronger, add 16 more repetitions with a "double beat" contraction at the fully abducted (open V) and adducted (closed V) positions. Use the added beat count to sustain a longer abdominal contraction.

Safety Tip: Perform this exercise only after you have mastered the other abdominal exercises and thereby strengthened your abdominals. If your abdominals are weak, you may find it difficult to avoid the excessive arch of your lower back (anterior pelvic tilt and corresponding spinal hyperextension) that can cause back injury.

PLANK

Equipment: Perform the Plank against the pool wall, or, for an intensified challenge, use two noodles held horizontally. For a highly advanced workout, use one noodle. Another way to increase the challenge is to use a kickboard; one with handles on each end works best.

Muscle Focus: This move strengthens your abdominal and torso-stabilizing muscles.

Starting Position: Stand facing the pool wall or with your hands on either side of the kickboard. Place your hands on the pool ledge at shoulder-width apart. Walk your feet back until your body forms a straight line. Place your feet somewhere between shoulder-width apart (beginner) or close together (advanced), with your toes on the pool floor, and flex at your ankle (figure a).

Action:

1. Contract the muscles of your torso, including your abdominals and buttocks, while keeping your lower spine in the neutral position. Keep your shoulder blades down and back (figure b).
2. Relax the contraction and repeat.
3. Repeat 8 to 16 times.

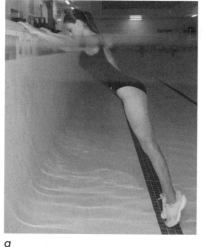
a

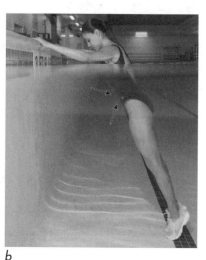
b

Variations:

- For variety, raise your hips to form a "V" with your body and then lower them again while contracting the stabilizing muscles of your torso.
- To increase the challenge of the Plank, lift one foot up off the pool floor, with a straight leg, and hold the contraction for several seconds. Repeat with the other leg. Avoid performing this exercise using a kickboard until you have very strong torso muscles that are ready for an advanced challenge.

Safety Tip: Avoid arching your lower back.

Back and Neck

When the abdominal muscles do a better job in stabilizing your body core, you have achieved an important component of back health. However, without balanced strength in the posterior (rear) elements of core stability, your body is imbalanced and injury is very likely to occur or become exacerbated. The moves in this section train your core muscles to work together for enhanced functional fitness. In fact, your abdominal muscles get another workout here, because they must work hard to stabilize your torso during the challenges posed by these moves. In addition to improving body alignment and stabilization, these moves enhance strength, strength through range of motion, and flexibility in the muscles that stabilize and move your upper back, midback, and lower back, as well as the muscles of your neck. Be sure to pay close attention to the safety tips and follow all of the exercise precautions, because your back and neck are two parts of your body that are the most vulnerable to injury caused by inappropriate technique. If you have had a challenge in the past with exercises designed to strengthen the spine, you may find the water moves described here much easier, more fun, and more comfortable to perform.

BIRD DOG POINT

MOVE
55

Muscle Focus: This move exercises your back muscles, stabilizes your pelvis, and strengthens your torso.

Starting Position: Stand facing the pool wall. Place your hands on the pool ledge at shoulder-width apart. Walk your feet back from the wall and bend at your hips. Place your feet shoulder-width apart, with your heels on the pool floor.

Action:

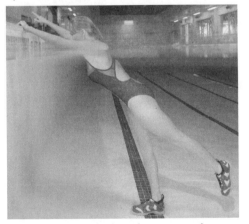

1. Contract your abdominal and buttocks muscles and lift your right arm to point straight overhead while you tighten your abdominals, squeeze your buttocks, and raise your left (opposite) leg behind you. Your arm, torso, and leg form a straight line; hold this position for several seconds. Bring your arm and leg back down.

2. Raise your left arm and right leg to form a straight line from your fingers through your torso to your toes; hold this position for several seconds. Bring your arm and leg back down.

3. Repeat 8 to 16 times.

Safety Tip: Keep your shoulder blades down and back throughout each step of the exercise. Remember to breathe deeply.

CAT BACK PRESS

Muscle Focus: This move exercises your back muscles.

Starting Position: Place your feet greater than shoulder-width apart, with your toes pointed slightly out to either side. Bend your knees and pull in your abdominals. Put your hands on your thighs midway between your knees and your hips (figure a).

Action:

1. Contract your abdomen and buttocks and press your navel up toward the sky, mimicking a cat stretching its back (figure b).
2. Flatten your back so that it is parallel to the pool floor.
3. Repeat 8 to 16 times.

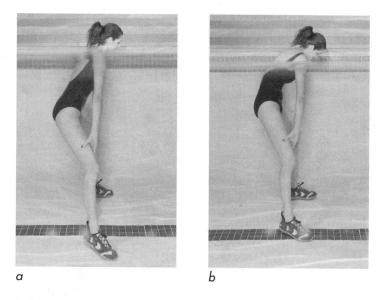

a   b

Variation: On the way down, press your navel toward the floor to make a swaybacked or U-shaped curve at your lower back.

Safety Tips: Move slowly and focus carefully on how each vertebra becomes part of the position change. This move improves flexibility and strength in the erector spinae muscles along the length of your spine and strengthens abdominal awareness.

Equipment: Use webbed gloves, water exercise bells, or paddles.

Muscle Focus: This move exercises the muscles of the shoulder's rotator cuff. Helps correct and prevent rounded shoulders.

Starting Position: Perform this exercise in chest- to shoulder-deep water. Stand with one foot in front of the other at shoulder-width apart or at a comfortable and stable distance apart. Contract your abdominal and buttocks muscles to brace your spine in the neutral position and stabilize your torso. Keep your chest lifted and your shoulder blades down and back. Bring both arms behind you, with your palms facing forward. Bend the arms at the elbow. Nestle your elbows into your waist. Keep your elbows stationary, behind your waist. Imagine that your upper arms are attached to your sides, and leave them in that position throughout the exercise. Your shoulders should be partly submerged.

Action:

1. Without moving your upper arms, press both hands to the left in an arc. Keep your elbows snugly positioned at your waist and avoid twisting your torso (figure a).
2. Press both hands to the right (figure b).
3. Repeat 8 to 16 times.

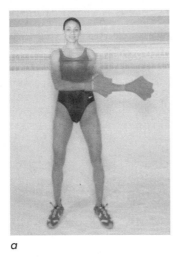
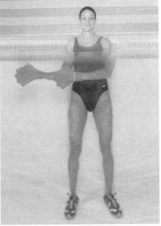

a   b

Variation: If you are using bells or paddles, perform this exercise using the wall for stability, with your back against the pool wall.

Safety Tip: For greater stability, perform this move with one arm at a time while you are holding on to the pool edge, with your side toward the wall. Be sure to keep your shoulder blades down and back.

SHOULDER SHRUG AND ROLL

Equipment: Use water exercise bells or paddles.

Muscle Focus: This move exercises the muscles of your upper back and shoulder.

Starting Position: Perform this exercise in chest- to shoulder-deep water. Stand with your feet shoulder-width apart and your arms at your sides. Contract your abdominal and buttocks muscles to brace your spine in the neutral position and stabilize your torso. Keep your chest lifted and your shoulder blades down and back. Bring both arms behind you; turn your palms to face forward.

Action:

1. Shrug your shoulders slowly by bringing them up toward your ears (figure *a*).

2. Slowly press your shoulders back and down (figure *b*). Repeat 8 times.

3. Roll your shoulders forward, up, back, and down. Repeat 8 times.

Safety Tip: Move slowly and smoothly; continue until any rubs, bumps, and crackles cease.

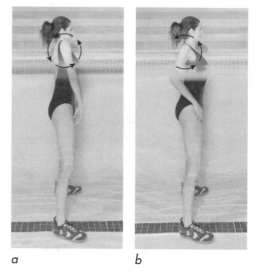

a   b

CHICKEN NECK BOB

Muscle Focus: This move exercises the muscles of the back of your neck and enhances your posture.

Starting Position: Place one foot slightly in front of the other to support a stable standing position. Bend your knees slightly and contract your abdominals. Stand upright, with your chest lifted and your shoulder blades back and down, your lower spine braced in the neutral position, with your abdominal and buttock muscles contracted.

Action:

1. Isolate the muscles of your neck (move your neck muscles only). Slowly bring your chin slightly forward; then contract the muscles on the back of your neck to press your head back, with your chin held level (neither lifted nor down) and your ears directly over your shoulders.

2. Repeat several times as you exhale on the muscle contraction and inhale on the muscle release.

3. Repeat 8 to 16 times.

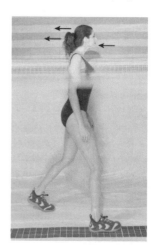

Safety Tips: Keep your chin level. Also, it is extremely important to avoid over-doing this exercise by extending or contracting beyond a controllable range of motion. In other words, your stabilization muscles must be doing their job to hold your neck, shoulders, and lower back in proper alignment. In fact, this is the main objective of the exercise: to train your stabilizers to maintain position through the range of front and back motion while you are improving the flexibility at your neck. Stronger, more flexible neck muscles can mean less neck pain and fewer headaches, as well as better posture.

Final Cool-Down

Finish every water exercise session with a Final Cool-Down Stretch sequence, as described in chapter 4, Warming Up and Cooling Down. If you skip the Final Cool-Down Stretches, your risk of soreness and injury increases significantly.

CHAPTER 7

Intensifying Workouts

Too often, people miss out on the benefits of regular exercise because they say to themselves, "I don't have enough time." Aquatic Exercise Association president Julie See describes aqua power and plyometrics aerobic exercises as the ideal time-saving solutions because they combine aerobic conditioning, fat burning, strength training, muscle endurance, flexibility enhancement, and a refreshing dip in the pool into one concentrated workout.

What makes aqua power and plyometric moves particularly beneficial is that they allow fit individuals, even those who have recuperated from injury, to accomplish more conditioning in less time. Power and plyometric techniques enable you to combine cardiorespiratory conditioning (aerobic exercise) with strength training and muscle toning through the use of exercises that elevate your heart rate into the aerobic working range while increasing the power capacity of your muscles and joints and toning your body. So in 1 hour, you can accomplish twice the endurance of aerobic exercise and toning activity possible in a regular format that calls for a separate toning section. However, to prevent injury, start by adding just a few power and plyometric moves to your program, performed at a slower pace, and then gradually replace your regular water aerobic moves with advanced moves one by one, speeding up the movement to raise intensity as you increase your fitness level in water. Don't take breaks between moves. Adjust intensity with pace and by adjusting resistance or eddy drag. Advance gradually and only within one of the four dimensions of the *FITT Principle* at a time: Frequency, Intensity, Type, or Time (time = duration). You will know you are ready to advance the challenge when you have been able to complete the existing level of challenge successfully for several weeks.

Powering Your Way to Fitness

Power and *plyometrics* are terms used to describe a particular type of advanced fitness technique. Power refers to "push-off" moves that use gravity, your body weight, and the floor to build strength and aerobic intensity. Power moves involve a variety of squatting exercises that make the muscles of your buttocks, hips, abdominals, and thighs work harder. The continuous action of these large muscle groups activates your aerobic energy system, improving cardiorespiratory endurance and burning fat stores. Properly performed, water squats also tone the muscles of your legs, hips, and buttocks by challenging your lower body to work against the resistance of your body weight and the viscosity of the water. Meanwhile, aquatic buoyancy and hydrostatic pressure take the pressure off your joints.

Plyometrics refers to "jump training" techniques that emphasize explosive leaping and bounding moves that can raise aerobic intensity and challenge your muscles. Plyometrics are powerful, controlled-impact jumps composed of explosive leaps. Plyometrics increase strength, endurance, coordination, reaction time, and aerobic and anaerobic capacity. Use of proper technique and preparation is essential for injury prevention.

When you can perform the Water Workout sequence illustrated in chapters 4 through 6 with proper form throughout, you have the basic level of fitness required to take on the challenges of more advanced techniques. Be sure to master the power moves before you move on to plyometrics. When you can maintain stabilized postures throughout the workout sequence, including power moves and all stretches, and finish without feeling fatigued, you have established the foundation required to succeed with plyometrics. With aquatic power and plyometric techniques for fitness training, you can make excellent use of your time and speed up your workout results. If you have built strong and flexible muscles and developed core strength, particularly in your torso, to protect yourself from injury, the power and plyometric moves described in this chapter can propel you into advanced levels of fitness. Water allows you to increase intensity in a protective atmosphere that is unavailable on land. The buoyancy of the water provides an ideal environment for these advanced fitness activities that are otherwise limited to sport-specific training and body building. Aquatic buoyancy supports the body structure, so it reduces stress on your joints during challenging moves. At the same time, the viscosity of the water increases resistance and enhances the toning, calorie burning, and strengthening effects of power and plyometric techniques.

For variety, alternate the power moves and plyometrics with regular aerobic moves. As you become more fit, this method challenges your cardiorespiratory system, enhances your fitness level, and gives you new ways to increase your intensity level to elevate your heart rate into the aerobic target zone. As you improve your execution of power moves, you can use them to maintain your target heart rate throughout your aerobics segment by using plyometric or regular jogs, jumping jacks, or slides for transitions between exercises.

Power and Plyometric Exercise Precautions

Because of the increased strain on the heart and body, people with joint pain, hypertension, or heart disease should seek guidance from a qualified medical or fitness professional before performing aqua power or plyometrics. Power and plyometric moves can be introduced comfortably and safely after you have developed a moderately high level of core strength, torso and limb stability, flexibility, and awareness of good body alignment.

When your fitness level has reached very advanced levels, perform your entire aerobic section or your entire fitness session with power and plyometrics for a highly challenging workout. Always begin with a complete warm-up and stretch before power and plyometrics and end with a thorough cool-down and stretch.

Use power and plyometrics to perform interval training, in which you escalate the aerobic intensity for a few minutes, return to a lower aerobic level, and then continue to alternate between the two levels throughout your workout. Including interval training from time to time can kick your fitness level up a notch. Practice the basics and perform them with complete control before you add these mighty moves to your program.

Using Proper Power Technique

You will be more comfortable if you start your power moves in waist-deep water. Before entering the water, practice your stance in front of a mirror (stand sideways) and compare your body position with figure 7.1. With practice, you should be able to balance so that you can "hover" over an imaginary chair—situated 1 or 2 feet (30 to 60 cm) behind you—while using the following techniques to protect your knees and spine. For squats, make sure that your knees are over your heels, not your toes, your buttocks are pressed back as if you were about to sit on a chair, your lower back is not arched, your chest is lifted, your shoulder blades are back and down, and your abdominal and buttocks muscles are contracted firmly to brace and protect your spine in a neutral position. Remember to breathe properly. Use the guidelines provided in the following list when performing power moves.

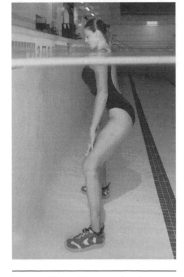

Figure 7.1 Correct body position for proper power technique.

Power Move Guidelines

- Warm up and then stretch all of the muscle groups beforehand to improve exercise efficiency and reduce risk of injury.

- Distribute your weight evenly around your body's center of gravity (usually located near your navel) and maintain the braced neutral position at your pelvis to help maintain proper body alignment. Strong abdominal muscles are a must.

- If your main objective is overall toning and endurance, limit the amount of resistance (use little or no resistance equipment) and do a higher number of repetitions. If you want to increase strength and develop more muscle shaping and definition, increase resistance and decrease repetitions.

- Always perform power moves slowly and with control, particularly when your are using resistance equipment.

- For good fitness results, squat to the depth that is comfortable (free of pain) and within your complete control, but with no more than 90 degrees of flexion at your knees. Practice and master strengthening move #40, the Wall Squat, from chapter 6, Strengthening and Toning, and power move #60, the Simple Squat, from this chapter before attempting to introduce additional power moves into your routine.

- To increase resistance with power moves: Add equipment such as the weighted X Vest, webbed gloves, or a Hydro Tone bell, Frisbee, or plastic dinner plate held gently but firmly in both hands at waist height, parallel to the floor, while you squat. Add resistance conservatively only after you have built a strong foundation of core strength and can perform the moves with complete control.

As you become more fit, add resistance equipment to increase the challenge of power moves in order to further enhance your fitness level. Use these techniques to strengthen the muscles of your buttocks, hips, and thighs and to improve the health of your knees and back. Squat with the weighted X Vest (figure 7.2a) to employ expertly designed technology that supports proper musculoskeletal alignment and biomechanics. Or use a Frisbee or plastic dinner plate (figure 7.2b) to displace water and created added resistance inexpensively. Be sure to keep your shoulder blades down and back and your chest lifted.

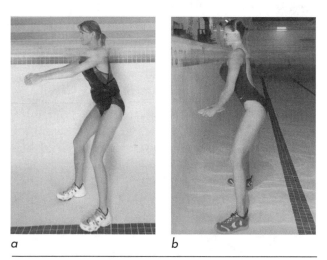

a   b

Figure 7.2 Equipment, used properly, increases resistance and builds strength and endurance.

Power Moves

SIMPLE SQUAT

Technique Tips: If you haven't tried this move before, give yourself time to refine the technique. Few people can manage a perfect squat on the first try or even after several attempts. Learning the basics of a squat is relatively simple, but mastering the technique takes time and practice. Proper technique always takes precedence over number of repetitions, depth of squat, and over adding resistance. Strive for the fullest range of motion (on raising and lowering) that you can manage without losing proper body form.

People who have never done squats before find themselves mainly focusing on not falling over: That is the body doing the work it needs to do to master the squat and all the stabilization and proprioceptive (balance and muscle control) skills needed to perform the squat successfully. As your body adapts, take the next steps to increase functional fitness by experimenting with squat stances. The reasons for trying out various stances is to find the one that is most advantageous for you or to challenge your body differently in order to enhance functional fitness.

There are two basic squat stances. Know what each stance involves. Every person is different, and there are many possibilities for variation. There are no hard and fast rules about which stance is right for you. For example, some people with longer legs find that they prefer a wider stance because it makes it easier for them to squat to their lowest controllable depth. In the wide stance, your feet are placed quite wide apart and your toes are often turned out. The wide stance emphasizes the work of your hamstrings (the back of your thighs), gluteals (buttocks), and hip joint, because hip extension (opening your hip joint into a standing position) provides much of the drive. As you lower into the squat, the range of motion at your hip joint eventually limits how far down you can squat. In the narrow stance, your quadriceps (the front of your thighs) work more. Those who are conditioning for skiing, for instance, may focus on a narrow stance squat in order to prepare the muscles for that specific challenge. Vary your stance in order to enhance functional fitness by strengthening your core and to tone your lower body.

Starting Position: In waist-deep water, stand with your feet about shoulder-width apart, with your knees pointing the same direction as your first and second toes and your feet pointed straight ahead or slightly turned out in a V.

(continued)

Action:

1. Imagine that there is a chair approximately 12 inches (30 cm) behind you; push your buttocks back and down toward the chair. Contract your buttocks as you squat, pull your abdominals in firmly, and balance your weight evenly front to back and left to right.

2. Tighten your buttocks and the backs of your thighs as you press yourself back into the upright starting position.

3. Repeat 16 to 32 times.

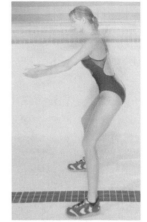

Variations:

- To increase your fitness level and improve toning results, change the distance between your feet and perform the squat in various stances, making the space wider or more narrow, as you become more proficient.

- Squat methods can also be modified to correct problems in technique. Knees caving inward can indicate, in part, a weakness in your hip abductors (the muscles that lift the leg to the side) or a pattern created by your performing the squat incorrectly over time. To change the pattern and focus on strengthening your hips, use this technique: Tie a piece of elastic tubing, an exercise band, or a length of string into a loop around your knees while standing. The loop should be tight enough around your knees so you can stand normally but loose enough that you have to press your knees outward to keep the band from falling down. Then execute the squat, making sure to press your knees outward throughout.

- Some knee pain results from weakness of the hip adductor (inner thigh) or vastus medialis (the part of the quadriceps closest to the inner thigh). If so, this squat modification may help: Squat as normal, but hold a Pilates ring or a water ball the size of a soccer ball between your knees. Focus on pressing inward as you squat. If you have any pain or dysfunction, consult a physician or physical therapist before using any of these fitness techniques.

Safety Tips: To protect your knee joints, make sure that your knees are behind your toes. Continually squatting with your knees protruding or pushing out over your toes strains the knee joint and creates or aggravates knee pain. Your ability to maintain this form determines how deeply you squat: Squat only as deeply as you can while still keeping your knees behind your toes. As you improve strength and flexibility, you may be able to squat more deeply with proper form. You actually achieve the advance in fitness when you challenge your muscles to maintain proper form during gradually increased challenges. Another important tip for knee protection is to avoid squatting to a depth that is below parallel with your knee joint (i.e., avoid squatting lower than a 90-degree angle at your knee). At this depth of squat, your thighs are parallel to the floor. Keep your chest lifted and your shoulder blades down and back to protect your spine: Avoid bending over or leaning forward at the waist in order to protect your back and hips from injury. Squat less deeply if you find yourself leaning forward or bending at the waist. Performed properly, Simple Squats enhance the health of your knees, back, and hips and create excellent improvements in your core strength. But if you perform them out of alignment and with improper body mechanics, they can create or exacerbate injuries.

SQUAT PRESS

Action: Repeat the action of the Simple Squat while employing all of the techniques and safety tips.

1. Straighten your arms down at your sides. As you squat, extend your arms from the shoulder out in front of you, scooping your palms toward the surface of the water. Keep your chest lifted.

2. As you rise, turn your hands around and press your palms down, returning your arms to your sides.

3. Repeat 8 to 32 times.

SQUAT KNEE LIFT

Action:

1. Perform the Squat Press (figure a).

2. As you rise, powerfully push up your left knee toward the surface of the water (figure b).

3. Squat again and, as your rise, powerfully push up your right knee toward the surface of the water.

4. Alternate right and left sequence for 8 to 32 repetitions.

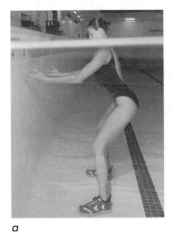

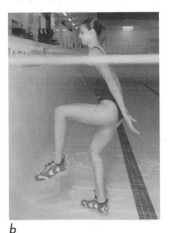

a   b

SQUAT KNEE CURL

Action:

1. Perform the Squat Press (figure *a*).
2. As you rise, extend at the hip and flex your left knee: Kick up your left heel toward your buttocks and draw your elbows back behind your waist (figure *b*).
3. Put your left foot down as you perform the Squat Press again.
4. As you rise, extend at the hip and flex your right knee: Kick up your right heel toward your buttocks and draw your elbows back behind your waist.
5. Repeat the sequence 8 to 32 times.

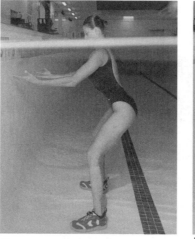 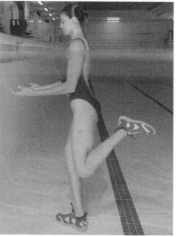

a   b

SQUAT SCISSOR LIFT

Action:

1. Squat and bend both arms at your elbow, pressing your palms toward your chest (figure *a*).
2. As you use your buttocks, thighs, and abdominals to press yourself into an upright position, lift your right leg out to the side. At the same time, straighten your arms and press them out to either side (figure *b*).
3. Bring your leg back in toward your body. At the same time, squat and bend both arms at your elbow, pressing your hands toward your chest.
4. Repeat, but press your left leg out to the side.
5. Repeat the sequence for 8 repetitions. Add more repetitions only when you are able to maintain excellent stability throughout each repetition.

Safety Tips: Maintain control by adopting the braced neutral position with firmly contracted abdominal and buttocks muscles. Keep your lifted leg low if you have a history of back pain.

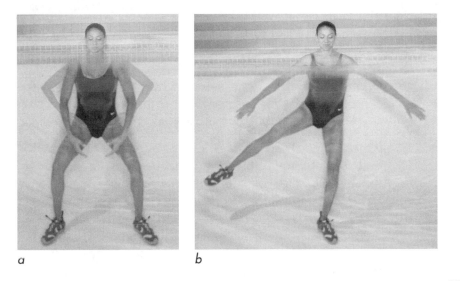

a   b

SQUAT STEP

Action:

1. Perform the Squat Press (figure a).
2. Squat and step out to the right at the same time (figure b). Press your arms out to the sides as you step out. Move from your hip and push sideways through the water powerfully to enhance the challenge of the move.
3. Bring your left leg in to meet your right leg as you stand upright, and bring your palms to your sides.
4. Repeat for 2 large, slower steps or 4 small, quicker steps.
5. Change direction and repeat the sequence: Step out with your left leg and draw your right leg in to meet your left leg. Repeat for 2 large, slower steps or 4 small, quicker steps.

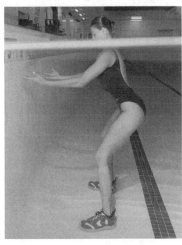 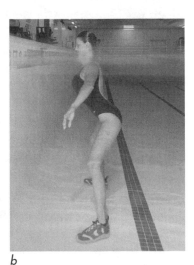

a   b

Stretch Tips to Improve Squat Technique

Several stretches help make proper squat technique easier and more effective. Execute stretching after a thorough warm-up. Perform these stretches as remedial work for the squat, both before and after you squat.

- **Squat Stretch.** The best range of motion or flexibility improvement activity for the squat is squatting itself. Perform the Squat Stretch by getting into the deepest squat you can achieve without losing proper form and staying in that position for a few seconds, letting your own weight assist the stretch. Ascend and repeat. If you do this stretch a few times every day or every workout, your muscles adapt within a few weeks and make the squat much easier to perform. You can also put on the weighted X vest for the Squat Stretch; the added weight helps increase the degree of stretch. To get a fuller hip stretch in this position, squat down with no weight on your back and, after you are at the bottom, use your elbows to push your knees outward. Hold for 5 seconds, ascend, and repeat as desired.

- **Stretch #9, Hamstring Stretch.** Tight hamstrings cause your lower back to round out at the bottom of the squat, straining your lower back. The most effective way to stretch the hamstring muscle group is to avoid toe touches and the Sit-and-Reach Stretch (which can tighten up your lower back) and perform instead the Hamstring Stretch, described in chapter 4, Warming Up and Cooling Down. Face the pool wall, place one foot on the pool wall and lengthen the back of your thigh while bending from your hip. The degree of hamstring flexibility determines how high you place your foot on the pool wall. If you cannot straighten your leg, your foot is too high. As you sink into the stretch, keep bending from your hip, not your waist, and push your buttocks back as you bring your upper body down, with your back flat, in a straight line.

- **Stretch #10, Deep-Muscle Hip, Thigh, and Buttocks Stretch.** Tight hips respond to the Deep-Muscle Hip, Thigh, and Buttocks Stretch. If you have not done this stretch before, you may not be able to stretch very far at first. As you progress, the farther forward you lean with a flat back, the more you feel the stretch in the outside of your hip. Because this is a deep stretch, you get better results when you breathe deeply and relax. Keep your front shin (standing leg) vertical, and avoid curling under at the pelvis. Press your buttocks back.

- **Calf Stretches #7 and 8.** Focus on these calf stretches if you find your heels rising as you lower your squat toward the floor.

- **Stretch #1, Outer-Thigh Stretch.** You can often alleviate pain on the outside of your knee by stretching your iliotibial band, which is a long strip of mostly connective tissue that runs down the outside of the thigh from the hip to the knee. Although the tissue spans the length of your thigh, it is most often felt in the knee area, outside and just above. Runners are especially likely to be familiar with the pain of iliotibial band irritation. You can relieve this knee pain by stretching and relaxing your hip abductor muscles, your gluteals, and your tensor fascia latae with the Outer-Thigh Stretch.

Plyometrics

Plyometrics is a term used to describe activities that enable a muscle to reach maximal force in the shortest possible time. Simply stated, plyometrics are exercises that involve a jumping or leaping movement and include skipping, bounding, jumping rope, hopping, lunges, and jump squats. A practical definition of plyometric exercise is a quick, powerful movement of lengthening and then shortening, called the stretch-shortening cycle—for example, jumping up and then drawing your knees to your chest and curling your torso into a ball.

Pushing your body upward explosively through water elevates your heart rate and trains your muscles to gain greater fitness using the principles of plyometrics. Pushing off the pool bottom and leaping—sideways, forward, straight up, or into a torso tuck—trains your muscles to marshal a great amount of force into one exertion. Repeating this exertion of force progressively overloads your muscles and cardiovascular system. Use plyometric techniques to activate your body's energy systems and musculoskeletal structure in order to

1. advance fitness level and improve body composition;
2. increase muscle power;
3. enhance sport performance;
4. challenge your body to improve balance, coordination, and agility;
5. tone and strengthen muscles;
6. increase healing and conditioning in the final stages of injury rehabilitation; or
7. add variety, challenge, and spice to your workout.

Muscles contract in three ways:

- An *eccentric* muscle contraction occurs when your muscle contracts and lengthens at the same time. One example of an eccentric muscle contraction is when you lower yourself from a chin-up position. Your biceps (upper-arm) muscle contracts and lengthens as you lower yourself from the chin-up bar.

- A *concentric* muscle contraction occurs when your muscle contracts and *shortens* at the same time. An example of a concentric muscle contraction is when you pull up into a chin-up position. Your biceps muscle contracts and shortens as you raise yourself up to the chin-up bar.

- An *isometric* muscle contraction occurs when your muscle contracts but does not change in length. An example of an isometric muscle contraction is when you hang from a chin-up bar with your arms bent at 90 degrees. Your biceps muscle contracts but does not change in length because you're not pulling up or lowering down.

The formal definition of plyometric exercise is one in which an eccentric (lengthening) muscle contraction is quickly followed by a concentric (shortening) muscle contraction. In other words, when a muscle is rapidly contracted while being lengthened and then immediately followed with a further contraction while being shortened. This process of contract and lengthen followed by contract and shorten is referred to as the *stretch-shortening cycle*.

Plyometric Exercises and Injury Prevention

Athletes often use plyometrics to develop power for sport performance, but few people realize how useful plyometrics can be in aiding injury prevention. Plyometric exercises tell the muscle to contract rapidly from a fully stretched position. At this position, muscles tend to be at their weakest point. By conditioning the muscle at its weakest point, at full stretch, the body is better prepared to handle this type of stress in a real, daily environment or during sport activities.

Plyometric Exercises and Injury Rehabilitation

An eccentric muscle contraction can require up to three times more force than a concentric muscle contraction. Therefore, plyometric exercises are essential in the final stage of injury rehabilitation in order to condition the muscles to handle the additional strain of eccentric (lengthening) contractions. When this final stage of the rehabilitation process is missing, the result is often reinjury, because the muscles have not been conditioned adequately to cope with the added force of eccentric muscle contractions. Eccentric muscle contractions are a common occurrence in day-to-day life and in sports and physical activity. Think about what is required in the following movements: lowering a small child to the ground after lifting him or her, reaching to catch a wide throw, or pushing a plate into place on the high shelf of a cabinet. If the body is not adequately trained to handle lengthening contractions following an injury, reinjury easily occurs.

Who Should Perform Plyometric Exercises?

Plyometrics are an advanced form of fitness and sport conditioning and can place a massive strain on unconditioned muscles, joints, and bones. Plyometric exercises should only be used by well-conditioned individuals and by those who have achieved effective rehabilitation results that have prepared them for a more advanced challenge. The water creates a more forgiving environment for plyometrics, making them safer for everyone, from the average person to the elite athlete. The key factor is to be sure that you have established a sound level of core strength before including plyometrics in your water workout sessions.

Plyometrics Precautions

There are several precautions to consider:

1. Intense, repetitive plyometric exercises are inappropriate for children or teenagers who are still growing.

2. You should develop a solid base of muscular strength and endurance, including torso core strength, before starting a plyometrics program.

3. A complete and thorough warm-up is required to prepare for the intensity of plyometric exercises.

4. Do not perform plyometric exercises on concrete, asphalt, or other hard surfaces. Grass is a good surface for plyometric exercises, but water is the best place to begin and enhances explosive movements and soft landings.

5. Body alignment and proper body mechanics are essential. As soon as you feel yourself getting fatigued or your form starts to deteriorate, stop. Consider hiring a qualified trainer or coach to guide you to develop proper technique.

6. Don't overdo it. Plyometrics activities are very intense. Give yourself plenty of rest between sessions, and skip a day between plyometric workouts; avoid doing plyometric exercises two days in a row, because your body needs 48 hours to complete the process of adaptation that strengthens muscles and tendons. Injury is likely if you do not allow enough time for this adaptation process to strengthen the tissues you have challenged.

Using Proper Plyometric Technique

When starting out, raise yourself up onto your toes, instead of leaping, until you feel comfortable pushing off the bottom of the pool. This helps you develop control over your body alignment technique and reduces your risk of injury caused by improperly performed leaps.

Start in waist- to chest-deep water, depending on what is most comfortable for you. Contract your abdominal and buttocks muscles firmly when you leap to avoid arching your lower back and overstraining your spinal stabilization structures. Always land with your knees bent; whenever possible, bring your heels all the way down to the floor.

Plyometrics Guidelines

- Before you add plyometrics to your workout, be sure that you have developed a good to excellent level of flexibility and strength. Especially essential is core strength of your torso, including strong abdominal and back muscles and all of the muscles that stabilize your pelvis, shoulder blades, and neck. Warm up and stretch all of the muscle groups before launching into power and plyometric moves in order to improve exercise efficiency and reduce risk of injury.

- Distribute your weight evenly around your body's center of gravity (usually somewhere near your navel).
- Land lightly, minimizing the intensity of impact with the floor.
- Use the braced neutral position and keep your body in proper alignment. Keep your back straight, your chest lifted, your shoulders back and down, and your ankles and knees in a bent (flexed) position; land with your knees behind your toes and your shoulders just behind your knees. When you elevate into a jump, be sure your abdominal and buttocks muscles are contracted firmly to brace your spine in neutral position and avoid hyperextension (inward curve) at your lower back.

Plyometric Moves

MOVE 66 — PETER PAN SIDE LEAP

Starting Position: Coil into a mini squat with your feet together to prepare for a powerful push-off. Start with your arms at your sides or straight out in front of you. (The squat position is shown in figure 7.1.)

Action:

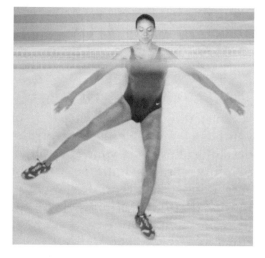

1. The basic move for a side leap is a step-apart side step. Imagine that you are leaping over a hurdle sideways, starting with your right leg. Press both arms out to your sides as you leap.

2. Land softly with your knees bent, and bring your left leg in to meet your right leg. Bring your palms down to your sides or bring them together out in front of you.

3. Repeat 4 times. Then repeat the sequence in the opposite direction, starting with your left leg.

HURDLE HOP

Starting Position: Coil into a mini squat with your feet together to prepare for a powerful push-off. Reach both arms out in front. Keep your shoulder blades down and back.

Action:

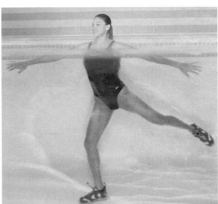

1. Lead with your right leg as you push off with your left leg in a forward leap. At the same time, press both palms out to the side in a breast-stroke motion.

2. Land on your right foot and bring your left foot forward to meet your right foot.

3. As you land, crouch again into the mini squat with your feet together.

4. Repeat a total of 4 times, leading with your right leg. Turn around and repeat 4 times, leading with your left leg. Add more sets as you become more proficient.

DOLPHIN JUMP

Starting Position: Start with your feet shoulder-width apart. Coil into a mini squat to prepare for a powerful push-off, with your arms outstretched at your sides at chest height. Keep your hands beneath the surface of the water.

Action:

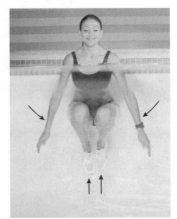

1. As you push off the bottom of the pool, tuck in your abdominals and bring your knees in toward your chest, using a very firm abdominal contraction. As you jump, thrust your palms in toward your sides, working from your shoulder joint.

2. Extend your legs, and land lightly with your knees bent; bring your hands apart, and push off again.

3. Repeat 8 to 32 times.

Variations:

- Push your palms toward one another under your thighs. Or perform facing the pool wall or ladder, and hold on with both hands.

- For a highly advanced version, stand away from the pool edge. Coil your body with your hands at shoulder height. As you push off, reach overhead, pushing toward the sky. As you land, bring your hands back to shoulder height. As you extend, keep a slight bend at your elbow to protect the joint and maintain a firm contraction with your abdominal and buttocks muscles in the braced neutral position to protect your spine.

PLYOMETRIC JACK

Starting Position: Coil into a mini squat with your feet together to prepare for a powerful push-off.

Action:

1. Push off the bottom and thrust your body upward using your buttock and thighs: Jump upward, drawing your knees up and coiling into a torso tuck (figure *a*). Then bring your legs wide apart, pressing both hands out to the sides (figure *b*). (Keep your hands underwater.)
2. Land lightly, with your feet wide apart, your knees slightly bent, and your heels down.
3. Push off the bottom and jump up, coiling into a torso tuck, using a very firm abdominal contraction. Then bring your legs back in and your knees up, as you bring your arms to your sides.
4. Touch down lightly and land with your feet together.
5. Repeat 8 to 16 times.

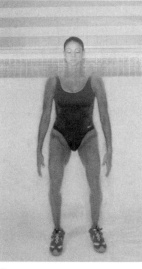
a

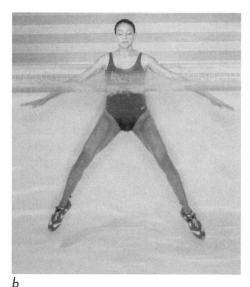
b

PLYOMETRIC SKI

Starting Position: Begin with your left foot in front and your right foot in back, firmly bracing your spine in the neutral position between your contracted abdominal and buttocks muscles. Reach forward with your right arm and back with your left arm (opposite of figure *b*).

Action:

1. Coil slightly and then push off the bottom and jump up (figure *a*). As you jump, draw your knees up, tuck your torso using a very firm abdominal contraction, and switch legs and arms (press your left foot back, your right foot forward, your right arm back, and your left arm forward). Focus to get your movement power from your hips, buttocks, and shoulders.

2. Land lightly, with your right foot forward, your left foot back, your left arm forward, your right arm back, and your knees slightly bent (figure *b*).

3. Repeat 8 to 16 times.

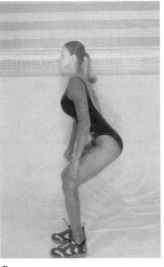
a

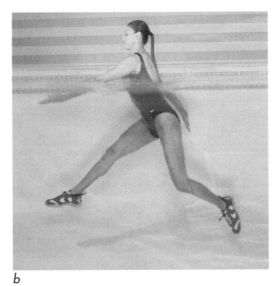
b

HIP, HOP, HURRAY!

Starting Position: Begin this highly advanced exercise with your feet shoulder-width apart and your hands raised to shoulder height (figure *a*).

Action:

1. Coil and crouch slightly, while contracting your abdominal and buttocks muscles very firmly.

2. Push off the bottom of the pool, while kicking your legs out to either side. At the same time, press your arms up overhead, just in front of your ears. Avoid locking your elbow joint as you straighten your arms. Maintain a firm contraction with your abdominal and buttocks muscles to strengthen and protect your back (figure *b*).

3. Bring your feet together and land lightly, with your knees slightly bent, in a mini squat; bring your heels all the way down. At the same time, bring your elbows down into the water. Keep your elbows bent.

4. Repeat 8 to 16 times.

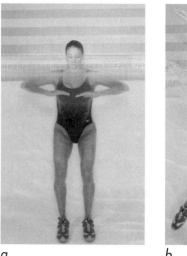 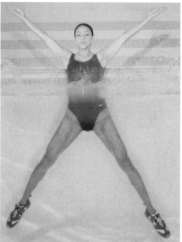

a   b

Variation: Stand in waist-deep water at the pool wall or ladder and perform the same move while holding on to the edge of the pool, pushing down with your arms as you jump up and bring your legs apart. Keep your legs pointing toward the bottom of the pool and your elbows slightly bent. This variation requires advanced upper-body and torso strength.

Safety Tip: Limit the number of repetitions to avoid the lack of control and the improper body mechanics that always accompany fatigue.

CHAPTER 8

Creating a Personal Water Workout

Every experienced exerciser, wellness coach and trainer knows the toughest challenge in keeping fit is getting started, setting meaningful goals and then keeping up the fitness habit. This chapter gives you powerful tools to get you started and keep you going. The step-by-step process walks you through identifying needs and preferences, barriers and solutions, and the decisions and plans you need to make in order to achieve your personal fitness goals. These basic strategies and techniques will help ensure a good start and enable you to successfully integrate water workouts as part of your healthy lifestyle.

- Create a plan that is right for your specific needs and circumstances.
- Make and sign a written commitment to yourself to make water fitness a priority.
- Create a time map that shows exactly where you will fit water workouts into your life, among the existing things you do on a daily and weekly basis.

The American College of Sports Medicine (ACSM) and American Heart Association (AHA) recommend that healthy adults under age 65 do a moderately intense cardio workout lasting 30 minutes, five days a week, or that they do a vigorously intense cardio workout for 20 minutes, three days a week. It is also suggested a person do eight to ten strength-training exercises, eight to twelve repetitions of each exercise twice a week.

Moderate-intensity physical activity means working hard enough to raise your heart rate and break a sweat, yet still being able to carry on a conversation. It should be noted that to lose weight or maintain weight loss, 60 to 90 minutes of physical activity may be necessary. The 30-minute recommendation is for the average healthy adult to maintain health and reduce the risk for chronic disease. Chapter 10 includes guidelines for adults over age 65 (or adults 50-64 with chronic conditions, such as arthritis).

If you like keeping records, a personal fitness journal can help you clearly identify your path and track your achievements. Or simply track your workouts on your calendar. A time map is a matrix you use to write down how you currently spend your time and to contemplate and decide how you would like to change your time and energy spent so that it more readily reflects your values, goals, and priorities. Table 8.1 illustrates the sample format of a time map. Tailor the matrix to your needs and include the time you wake up, the time you go to sleep, eating time, work time, commuting time, fitness time, play time, rest time, and any other activities or processes. And, of course, when you modify your map, be sure to include your water workouts!

Fill out your time map based on how you currently spend your time during an average week. Then explore areas where you may be spending more time on items of lower priority—cut back that time, carving out time for higher priority items. Reorganize your schedule as needed, and use the new-found time to build in a regularly scheduled time for your water workouts.

You will have more success with your water workouts when you follow these progressive steps to creating a water workout sequence that matches what will work best for you:

1. Identify your current fitness profile.
2. Understand your "fitness personality."
3. Establish realistic fitness goals.
4. Think about the barriers and obstacles that have held you back from being successful at fitness in the past and explore how to overcome them.
5. Choose first steps that are immediately achievable and help build fitness success.
6. Make a plan for success with your long-term goals.
7. Start to build new fitness habits one step at a time.
8. Approach roadblocks and setbacks with imagination, openness, and a new perspective on the steps it takes to be successful.
9. Celebrate your successes and reward yourself for making progress.

Use the forms in the appendix of this book to complete the steps to creating a water workout sequence that is right for you. If you photocopy the forms, you can fill them out again at some time in the future as you increase your fitness level or as your needs and goals change. Take it step by step; there's no need to complete the whole series at one time. It may be better to work on parts of the profile and planning forms, think about your responses, and then return later to work on them again. As you begin to apply what you discover from going through the process, take your time and try one or two of the ideas

Table 8.1 Time Map

Time/Day	Sunday	Monday	Tuesday	Wednesday	Thursday	Friday	Saturday
6:00 a.m.							
7:00 a.m.							
8:00 a.m.							
9:00 a.m.							
10:00 a.m.							
11:00 a.m.							
12:00 noon							
1:00 p.m.							
2:00 p.m.							
3:00 p.m.							
4:00 p.m.							
5:00 p.m.							
6:00 p.m.							
7:00 p.m.							
8:00 p.m.							
9:00 p.m.							
10:00 p.m.							

and recommendations. Then come back and refer to the planning tool again to decide what to add or eliminate next.

Refining Your Water Workout Plan

Identify your goals and methods by using the resources in this chapter and in the appendix and by referring to the segments throughout the book that the planning process has identified as relevant. As you build new fitness habits, remember the wise words of wellness professional Murray Banks of Peak Performance: "Inch by inch it's a cinch. . . Yard by yard it's too hard." If you are patient but persistent and you change just one small step at a time and learn from your setbacks, your efforts will be rewarded with success.

Ingredients for a Successful First Water Workout

Perhaps you are a water baby, like the author, and are very familiar with how your body moves in the water. On the other hand, when you try your first water workout you may feel like you are in a foreign environment, a "fish out of water." An important key to getting the most out of your first time is to tune in to how comfortable, satisfying, and invigorating water workouts can be. Follow these basic starter tips for success:

1. Focus on becoming more familiar with how your body moves in water and how your control of your movements develops with a bit of practice and concentration. As you continue to engage in water workouts regularly, your systems adapt to the unique balance and agility aspects of the aquatic environment and your control of your movements becomes reflexive and automatic.

2. Listen to how your body responds to the challenge. Judge how long to continue exercising and determine how hard to push based on how you feel. During the aerobic and muscle toning segments, you will know that it's time to change what you are doing when you feel fatigue coming on. During your aerobic section, fatigue is a signal for you to begin the gradual descent into an aerobic cool-down. During muscle toning, fatigue or loss of postural control indicates that it's time to change to another exercise. If you are still charged up after 8 repetitions, complete about 8 more but never continue to exercise once you feel fatigue or loss of proper body alignment. To do so greatly increases your risk of injury and illness.

3. If you are just starting out, begin slowly. Build the challenge gradually, over weeks and months. There is absolutely no need to over-push yourself when you begin any new exercise program. Your body must adapt gradually to the introduction of new exercise. So take it easy the first several times you work out. Get to know your muscles and how they work together to move your joints and stabilize your body: Develop "body awareness." When you become adept at controlling your muscle movements and breathing, you can begin to intensify your program along the *FITT principle* (Frequency, Intensity, Type, and Time; see chapter 3, Understanding the Phases of a Water Workout, for details). Increase very gradually in *one category at a time*, and allow a week or more between each type of increase for your body to adapt to the new challenge. For instance, if your aerobic section is 10 minutes long, increase it to 11 minutes the next week, 12 minutes the following week, and so on until you reach your objective. If you are exercising three times a week and wish to add a day, exercise four times a week for a shorter period each time for several weeks, and then gradually increase the duration. If you plan to increase muscle strengthening intensity with equipment, start out with no equipment until you are stable, steady, and strong with your water resistance exercises and body positioning. Then build your intensity gradually, by adding equipment or increasing the force or speed of your movements.

4. Before you begin your first water workout, check with your doctor to find out if you need medical clearance before beginning to exercise.

5. Consult the section called Tailor Workouts for Special Needs in chapter 10, Special Workouts for Special Needs, to customize your workout to address any particular considerations that are important for you.

6. Reread the Injury Prevention Checklist on pages 19-23.

7. Make sure that the temperature of the water in your pool is about 78 to 86 degrees Fahrenheit (26 to 36 degrees Celsius).

8. Be sure that someone is nearby in case you need assistance.

Table 8.2 provides a Basic Starter Water Workout sequence. Follow it the first several times you work out in the pool, tailoring it to your changing needs as you improve your fitness. Refer to the descriptions in chapters 4, 5, and 6 for more detailed instructions on each exercise.

Table 8.2   Basic Starter Workout: 35-45 minutes

Thermal Warm-Up (5 minutes)	Perform this Thermal Warm-Up sequence twice. Start slowly and build very gradually.
	Move #1 Water Walk: 30 seconds
	Move #2 Pedal Jog: 30 seconds
	Move #9 Heel Jacks: 8 times
	Move #10 Alternate-Leg Press-Back: 8 times
	Move #12 Snake Walk: 1 minute
Warm-Up Stretch (5 minutes)	Hold each stretch position for 10 seconds.
	Stretch #1 Outer-Thigh Stretch
	Stretch #2 Lower-Back Stretch With Ankle Rotation
	Stretch #4 Shin Stretch and Shoulder Shrug
	Stretch #5 Inner-Thigh Step-Out
	Stretch #6 Hip Flexor Stretch
	Stretch #7 Straight-Leg Calf Stretch
	Stretch #8 Bent-Knee Calf Stretch
	Stretch #9 Hamstring Stretch
	(Repeat previous sequence for the other side of your body.)
	Stretch #10 Deep-Muscle Hip, Thigh, and Buttocks Stretch
	Stretch #11 Full Back Stretch
	Stretch #12 Midback Stretch
	Stretch #13 Elbow Press-Back
	Stretch #14 Shoulder Roll and Chest Stretch
	Stretch #15 Chest Stretch
	Stretch #16 Upper-Back Stretch
	Stretch #17 Torso and Shoulder Stretch
	Stretch #18 Shoulder and Upper-Arm Stretch
	Stretch #19 Safe Neck Stretch
Aerobic Exercises (10-15 minutes)	In this section, start slowly, build gradually, and then gradually decrease intensity.
	Move #1 Water Walk: 1 minute
	Move #2 Pedal Jog: 30 seconds
	Move #9 Heel Jacks: 8 times
	Move #10 Alternate-Leg Press-Back: 8 times

(continued)

Table 8.2 *(continued)*

Aerobic Exercises *(continued)*	Move #13	Step Wide Side: 8 times in each direction
	Move #14	Hydro Jacks: 8 times
	Move #15	Cross-Country Ski: 16 times
	Move #12	Snake Walk: 1 minute
	Move #26	Aqua Ski: 10-30 seconds
	Move #27	Floating Side Scissors: 10-30 seconds
	Move #28	Back Float Kick and Squiggle: 10-30 seconds
	Move #29	Vertical Frog Bob: 10-30 seconds
	Move #30	Vertical Flutter Kick: 10-30 seconds
	Move #32	Bicycle Pump: 10-30 seconds
	Move #12	Snake Walk: 1 minute
	Move #13	Step Wide Side: 8 times right, 8 times left
	Move #10	Alternate-Leg Press-Back: 8 times
	Move #9	Heel Jacks: 8 times
	Move #1	Water Walk: 1 minute
	Move #2	Pedal Jog: 30 seconds
Muscle Strengthening and Toning Exercises (5-10 minutes)	Move #34	Outer- and Inner-Thigh Scissors: 8 times
	Move #35	Forward-and-Back Leg Glide: 8 times per side
	Move #39	Pivoted Dip: 4 times per side
	Move #40	Wall Squat: 8 times, 2 or 3 sets
	Move #42	Calf Lift: 8 times
	Move #44	Chest and Upper-Back Glide: 8 times
	Move #48	Pivoted Shoulder Press: 8 times
	Move #49	Side Arm Pump: 4 times
	Move #50	Upper-Arm Curl: 8 times
	Move #58	Shoulder Shrug and Roll: 4 times each
	Move #51	Wall-Sit Crunch and Rock-Belly Crunch: 8 times
	Move #52	Floating Curl: 8 times (avoid this one if it irritates your neck)
	Move #55	Bird Dog Point: 8 times
	Move #56	Cat Back Press: 8 times
Final Cool-Down Stretches (10 minutes)	Repeat the entire Warm-Up Stretch sequence, but hold each stretch for 20 seconds.	

Follow this sequence the first several times you work out in the pool. Before you start, familiarize yourself with the specific instructions for each exercise and stretch.

Workouts Tips for Specific Body Types

Have you ever wondered why some people seem to get slim and toned after just a few weeks of exercise, while others have to follow the identical fitness and nutrition practices for many months to achieve the same results? Is everyone potentially a slender model or muscular body builder? No. Here's why.

There are three main hereditary body types: ectomorph, endomorph, and mesomorph (see figure 8.1). Most people generally fit into one category or another or have traits of two types mixed together. If you're unsure of your body type, identify the traits you had as a child or teenager, before your lifestyle may have disguised your true genetic characteristics.

Ectomorphs tend to be long and lanky. They are small boned, with limbs longer in relation to their trunk. Muscles are not well defined. Ectomorphs are not likely to increase much in muscle size or bulk, but they may have an easier time with weight control than people with an endomorphic body type. People with long, thin muscles are more likely to experience back pain than people with other body types.

Endomorphs are rounded and curvy. The body tends to be pear shaped, with soft, rounded shoulders and wider, padded hips. Limbs are shorter relative to the trunk. People with an endomorphic body type often have a slower metabolism and have a tougher time losing weight.

The person with the mesomorph body type builds muscle easily. Mesomorphs are broader at the shoulders and hips, narrower at the waist. Their well-defined musculature make them appear fit even when they don't

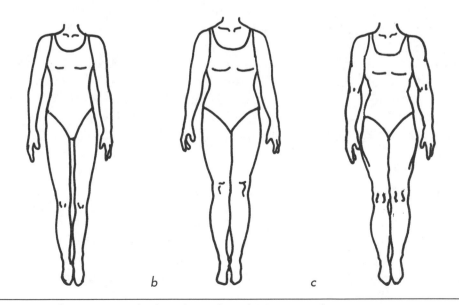

a   b   c

Figure 8.1   The (a) ectomorph, (b) endomorph, and (c) mesomorph.

exercise. Their lack of flexibility can expose them to the risk of injury to the back, neck, and lower leg. They have a speedy metabolism, which is related to having denser muscle tissue. Like all of the types, mesomorphs put on weight if they eat more calories than they burn. When they add extra weight, people with mesomorphic body type take on the "apple" shape associated with heart disease.

Many people have a combination of body types. "Endo-mesomorphs" have naturally stronger muscles along with higher ratios of body fat and tend to carry more weight in the hips and thighs. "Ecto-mesomorphs" are long, thin, and wiry, with well-defined muscles. "Endo-ectomorphs" tend to carry more weight in the hips and thighs, although they are long limbed and small boned and have long and slender upper bodies and may lack upper-body strength.

Each body type has advantages and disadvantages. The point is to identify your own characteristics and develop realistic and appropriate fitness objectives. You look and feel your best when you are healthy and fit, with well-aligned body posture and higher energy. Choose an exercise plan based on your own characteristics and your personal fitness objectives.

Ectomorphs

Follow the Basic Starter Water Workout program, but focus on building muscle strength and flexibility. Gradually add increased resistance by using water exercise equipment, as described in chapter 2, Preparing for Water Workouts. Emphasize strengthening for your abdominals and trunk to prevent lower-back problems. Concentrate carefully on stretching techniques to improve flexibility in your hips, thighs, buttocks, back, neck, and torso.

The ectomorph's muscles get somewhat stronger with conditioning but require more effort and time to appear firm and toned. A thin body can still be proportionally high in body fat (overfat), so ectomorphs need to pursue aerobic training to maintain good overall health. Gradually strengthen your abdominals and trunk and work carefully on torso and lower-body flexibility to combat susceptibility to problems in your lower back and neck.

Endomorphs

You can improve your body composition and speed up your metabolism by following the Basic Starter Water Workout program and concentrating on the recommendations for weight control described in the section in this chapter called Tone Up and Lose Weight. Endomorphs can be prone to injury from impact stress. It is essential that you protect your joints through low-impact exercise, so water exercise is a method of choice. As you become more fit, strive to extend your aerobic section to 45 minutes or more; that is the point at which a greater percentage of calories burned comes from body fat stores versus the quick energy of glycogen in your muscles. Keep the aerobic intensity moderate in order to extend the length of your aerobic section.

Body toning and weight control can be more challenging for people with this genetic body type because of their higher ratios of fat to lean tissue (body composition). Aerobic conditioning and resistance or weight training can improve body composition, metabolism, and muscle definition. Changing your body composition to one with a higher ratio of lean to fat tissue helps you achieve and maintain weight loss over the long haul.

Mesomorphs

Mesomorphs frequently have taut, firm muscles. Tight, tense muscles lead to pain and discomfort and can limit your mobility, especially later in life. Lengthen the final stretch and flexibility section of your routine to 10 or 15 minutes to relax your tight muscles. Work on improved aerobic endurance for functional stamina and cardiovascular health; mesomorphs can be prone to heart and circulatory ailments. So strive for workouts each week, on most days of the week, that include a full aerobic section and that conclude with a relaxing flexibility segment. You may want to develop further your naturally muscular physique by gradually increasing the resistance used during Strengthening and Toning Moves.

Mesomorphs respond quickly to resistance training and become firm and toned with less effort than ectomorphs or endomorphs. The mesomorphic body type is quicker to drop fat, which generally collects around your abdomen. However, the mesomorphic body type usually needs to work on flexibility to relax tight muscles and on aerobic conditioning to improve cardiorespiratory endurance and stamina. Because mesomorphs look fit even if they are out of shape, some may be less motivated to exercise and that often leads to the gradual accumulation of abdominal fat.

Tone Up and Lose Weight

In the United States, more than 68 percent of people are overweight or obese. The phenomenon exists in many other countries of the world as well. Because weight management is a priority for a growing number of people and for society as a whole, this section is devoted to how to use water workouts and other lifestyle techniques to be successful with weight control. Use the following tips for success with weight management.

Build the duration and intensity of your aerobic exercise gradually, over a period of several months, and increase your muscle resistance training gradually. You burn off excess body fat aerobically. To focus your efforts on weight control, to lose weight, and to keep it off, increase your lean body mass and reduce your fat mass. Aerobic endurance activities can train your body to become a more efficient fat burner. Muscle strengthening can build your lean tissue mass. Lean tissue burns more calories, even when you are at rest. So include muscle strength and endurance exercises not only to tone up, but also to increase the rate at which you burn calories all of the time.

Chart your progress by measuring inches. Avoid using the scale, and instead measure waist circumference every 4 to 8 weeks to chart your progress. A handful of muscle weighs much more than a handful of fat, so the scale can be misleading. A pound of muscle takes up much less room than a pound of fat; that is why two people who weigh 160 lbs—one muscular and fit and the other with a high body fat ratio—look completely different. The muscular person has significantly smaller circumferential measurement at the waist and many other parts of the body, as well as more energy, confidence, and vitality!

Build the frequency of workouts gradually. If you have been sedentary, start by exercising every other day. Build up to five days a week as you increase your fitness level. Eventually, make physical activity and exercise a part of nearly every day of the week. In order to change your body composition by increasing lean tissue, include strengthening and toning in at least two of your workouts each week. A good rule of thumb for strength training is to work the muscle group every *other* day. If you alternate muscle groups, you can perform resistance training every day, but avoid working the same muscle group two days in a row. When starting out, focus on strengthening your torso, especially your abdominal, back, and buttocks muscles. If you want to encourage greater fat burning during workouts, gradually lengthen the duration of your aerobic activity rather than push for the highest possible intensity. High-intensity aerobic activity often brings on fatigue and produces injuries unless you are extremely fit.

For the best results, combine your fitness program with a healthy eating plan. Always eat breakfast, within one hour of waking up; gradually reduce your intake of empty calories from fatty foods, such as fried foods and processed meats; and cut down on foods with added sugars. (Read labels carefully: Sugar is added in many forms.) Eat fewer white potatoes, fewer refined grains, such as white flour, and more whole grains. Eliminate trans fat (hydrogenated and partially hydrogenated fat), and drink lots of fluids, especially water. Cut no more than approximately 500 calories from your daily intake or else you may trigger your body to slow its metabolism.

To stoke your metabolism and avoid getting overly hungry, eat three meals and two snacks or mini meals a day, spacing your food throughout the day. Eat at least two-thirds of your calories or servings by midday. Stop eating two or three hours before bedtime.

Use this portion control guideline, based on the new Food Guide Pyramid. Every day, eat these portions, spread throughout the day:

- **Grains.** Eat six servings, at least three of which are whole grain: serving size, the palm of your hand; flakey grains, twice the size of your palm.

- **Vegetables.** Eat five or more servings: serving size, the palm of your hand; leafy vegetables, twice the size of your palm.

- **Fruits.** Eat two servings: serving size, the size of your fist. Eat whole fruit to get more fiber and to absorb the sugar more slowly than with processed fruits.

- **Oil.** Eat six to ten servings: serving size, the tip of your largest finger, or approximately a teaspoon. The best sources are extra virgin olive oil, walnut oil, or sesame oil. Eating enough healthy fats is very important to good nutrition. Read labels, especially on baked goods and processed foods, and avoid transfat and partially hydrogenated vegetable oils. Unless they are transfat free, steer clear of most margarine and shortenings.

- **Protein.** Eat two servings: serving size, the palm of your hand. Protein sources include fish, poultry, legumes or beans (e.g., kidney, garbanzo, pinto, black beans), nuts (especially walnuts and almonds), lean cuts of red meat (sparingly), eggs (sparingly). Eggs, fish, nuts, poultry, and meat also contain fat.

- **Water.** Drink eight servings: serving size, two fists. You generally take in about two water servings a day if you consume all of the recommended servings of fruits and vegetables; get the rest by drinking fluids that are not diuretic. Caffeinated drinks and drinks with citrus are diuretic and therefore stimulate the loss of fluids from the system. Drink more water when you are very active in hot weather. If you don't like water, try water with a splash of unsweetened fruit juice.

- **Calcium.** Eat three servings. Size varies. Eat more low-fat, less full-fat foods containing calcium: one slice of low-fat cheese, one-half cup of low-fat cottage cheese, one cup of low-fat yogurt, eight ounces of enriched soy or rice milk or cow's milk, one-half cup of enriched tofu, or one cup of green, leafy vegetables.

- **Discretionary calories.** As a discretionary allowance, include 132 to 512 calories per day, depending on your activity level, gender, and goals. Discretionary allowance includes solid fat, cookies, donuts, pastries, crackers containing fat, candy, soda, chips, meats, butter, whipped cream, cream cheese, half and half, or sour cream. One medium-sized cookie contains 100 calories. Some plant fats are also in the solid fat category: Palm oil, palm kernel oil, coconut oil, and cocoa butter. Fat contains about 100 calories per tablespoon. Fats contain about twice as many calories per gram compared to other foods. Healthy fat (see oil and fat) plays a critical role in healthy eating and supports many bodily processes. You can use your discretionary calories by eating from any of the other food groups.

Don't try to tackle everything at once; take it step by step, one step at a time. Select one *small* change by making it part of your lifestyle until you are comfortable with it. Then take the next small step for which you feel ready.

Adding Variety to Your Workouts

What makes variation so important to fitness success? The reasons stem from basic fitness principles and factors for change in health behavior. First, people get bored with doing the same thing over and over again, day after day, and variety keeps interest levels recharged. Second, the body requires various challenges from time to time in order to make improvements in fitness level, for instance, the challenge of interval training to prompt new adaptations that improve the condition of your cardiovascular system. Third, the fitness principle referred to as cross-training calls for making changes in the type of impact shock or in methods of resistance in order to avoid or overcome repetitive stress injuries. An example of modifying impact shock is when you change from shallow end aerobic moves that require a mild amount of impact with the pool bottom to flotation exercise that eliminates impact shock completely. Another example is when you alternate walking or running on land with bicycling. Variety helps prevent and overcome roadblocks that can get in the way of maintaining your fitness program or making the progress you aspire to in your lifelong journey toward fitness and wellness.

Water workouts present an excellent opportunity for cross-training fun for people who are already advanced in their fitness capabilities. The following sequence in table 8.3 combines many of the most advanced techniques that are sure to give your body, mind, and spirit a heightened challenge and a new twist on your workouts. For a sensual variation that is sure to stimulate your funky inner nature, challenge your aerobic fitness, strengthen your core, and tweak your balance and coordination, try the Water Yoga Booty Ballet sequence found in table 9.1.

Table 8.3 Sample Advanced Water Workout

Thermal Warm-Up (5 minutes)	Move #82	Circle the Drum
	Move #83	Embracing the Moon
	Move #84	Kick Back and Front
	Move #85	Arm Circling
	Move #86	Scoop the Earth
	Move #87	Pat High on Horse: Pat and Pull
	Move #88	Parting the Wild Horse's Mane
Warm-Up Stretch (also enhances balance and strength) (5 minutes)	Move #94	Salutation to the Sun
	Move #95	Bow and Arrow Warrior Pose
	Move #96	Flamingo or Superman Pose
	Move #97	Half Lotus
	Move #98	Half Moon
	Move #99	Tree Pose
	Move #100	Triangle Extended-Angle Pose
	Stretch #3	Front-of-Thigh Stretch
	Stretch #7	Straight-Leg Calf Stretch
	Stretch #8	Bent-Knee Calf Stretch
	Stretch #9	Hamstring Stretch
	Stretch #10	Deep-Muscle Hip, Thigh, and Buttocks Stretch
	Stretch #11	Full Back Stretch
	Stretch #17	Torso and Shoulder Stretch
	Stretch #18	Shoulder and Upper-Arm Stretch
Aerobic and Plyometrics Moves (30 to 45 minutes) **Create combinations and repeat moves as desired.**	Move #15	Cross-Country Ski
	Move #13	Step Wide Side
	Move #14	Hydro Jacks
	Move #17	Jump Forward, Jump Back
	Move #18	Mountain Climbing
	Move #19	Ski and Jack Combo
	Move #20	Mogul Hop
	Move #23	Lunge and Center
	Move #24	Lunge Kick Square
	Move #25	Jump Twist
	Move #26	Aqua Ski
	Move #31	Floating Mountain Climb (with flotation)
	Move #37	Runner's Stride (with flotation)

(continued)

Table 8.3 *(continued)*

Aerobic and Plyometrics Moves (30 to 45 minutes) **Create combinations and repeat moves as desired.** *(continued)*	Move #66	Peter Pan Side Leap
	Move #67	Hurdle Hop
	Move #68	Dolphin Jump
	Move #69	Plyometric Jack
	Move #70	Plyometric Ski
	Move #71	Hip-Hop Hooray!
Anaerobic Power and Strength	Move #60	Simple Squat
	Move #61	Squat Press
	Move #62	Squat Knee Lift
	Move #63	Squat Knee Curl
	Move #64	Squat Scissor Lift
	Move #65	Squat Step
	Move #75	Kickboard Climb
	Move #89	Forward Jab
	Move #90	Cross Jab
	Move #91	Shin Block
	Move #92	Knee Strike
	Move #93	Front Kick From Rear Leg or Front Leg
Core Strength Builders	Move #101	Saw
	Move #73	Noodle Sidewinder
	Move #74	Noodle Ring
	Move #102	Half-Moon Tightrope Touch
	Move #103	Leg Circles
	Move #104	Diagonal Bicycle Pump
	Move #51	Rock-Belly Crunch (Wall Sit Crunch away from wall)
	Move #105	Plank and Press
Range of Motion: Release for Muscles of the Spine.	Move #106	Otter
Cool-Down Stretch		Repeat the Warm-Up Stretch sequence, but hold each stretch longer, for 20 seconds. To increase the challenge perform the stretches without touching the pool wall.

CHAPTER 9

Adding Splash to Workouts

The best way to sustain your workouts over the long term is to introduce new techniques continually and to spice things up with variety. Variation keeps you interested, challenges your body differently, and increases fitness. Use this chapter to dig for valuable workout gems and different ideas to recharge your workouts with renewed excitement. Choose from down-home fun with Water Country Line Dancing, the grace and energy of Water Tai Chi, the stress-busting power of Water Kickboxing, the peace and fulfillment of Water Yoga, the core strength of Water Pilates, or the body-tingling funk of Water Yoga Booty Ballet.

Creative Water Workouts

Creativity fuels motivation and helps maintain your interest in continuing to work out on a regular basis. Introduce these moves to challenge your body, mind, and spirit in ways that can enhance your physical fitness and nourish your overall well-being. Step out of the box of what you are used to. Let your imagination, interests, and personality guide you to introduce these moves into your routine or to create a whole new sequence. Create combinations that stimulate your senses and keep you moving along on your fitness journey.

Noodle Moves

The genius of the inexpensive water noodle is in the freedom of movement made possible by its simple, flexible design. Stir up some fun and achieve enhanced musculoskeletal stabilization, improved back health, tighter abdominals, and a stronger, toned-up torso with these Noodle Moves. Insert these moves into your water workout in nearly any body of water to achieve a combined aerobic conditioning and torso-toning segment. Focus on these conditioning moves after a light warm-up and stretch, and follow them with a series of stretches that include those for your torso, back, hips, and thighs. There are long noodles and shorter noodles; use the shorter ones if you plan to sit on them for flotation. Tip: Save money by buying inexpensive long noodles where toys are sold and cutting them to the desired length.

The section on Water Pilates starting on page 187 contains additional Noodle Moves.

MOVE 72 — WATER BUG BELLY CRUNCH

Muscle Focus: This move works your abdominal muscles.

Starting Position: This noodle crunch is performed with the noodle behind your upper back and under your arms; your arms should be outstretched to your sides at shoulder level and resting on the noodle. Start with the bottoms of your feet together and your knees slightly bent, in a seated position, with a partial abdominal crunch (partially contracted abdominals). Imagine your abdominal or belly muscles as an accordion.

Action:

1. With your heels together, tighten or contract your abdominal muscles to "close the accordion," as you draw your knees up and out at the same time.
2. Straighten your legs as you press your feet back out in front of you (open the accordion). Maintain a partial contraction of your abdominal muscles.
3. Inhale at the start, exhale as you contract, and inhale as you lengthen.
4. Repeat 8 to 32 times.

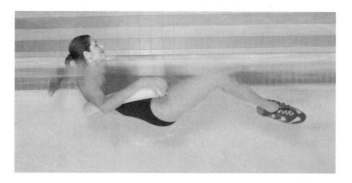

Variation: The Noodle Side Crunch works your oblique abdominals, on your sides. Start with your feet together, in a seated position, and your legs relatively straight, with a slight abdominal contraction. Turn your hips slightly to the right and shorten the distance from your rib cage to your hip. Repeat 4 to 16 times. Turn your hips slightly to the left and repeat 4 to 16 times.

NOODLE SIDEWINDER

Muscle Focus: This aerobic move works the mover and stabilizer muscles of your torso, including your abdominals, obliques, serratus anterior, quadratus lumborum, and erector spinae (front, back, and sides of your torso).

Starting Position: This noodle toner is performed with the noodle behind your upper back and under your arms; your arms should be outstretched to your sides at shoulder level and resting on the noodle. For added stability and slightly increased resistance, grasp a second noodle held horizontally in front with both hands. Keep the abdominals contracted firmly throughout the motion.

Action:
1. Pedal your legs as if you were on a bicycle.
2. Contract the muscles in your right side to bring your feet out to the side. Use the muscles of your side as you would in a Side Crunch. The pedaling motion in this position challenges the oblique muscles on both sides of your abdomen, so use them and your frontal abdominals (rectus abdominus) to maintain stability as you pedal your legs in a circular motion.
3. Keep pedaling as you spin around in a circle. Continue for 10 to 20 seconds.
4. Repeat on your left side, spinning around in the opposite direction.

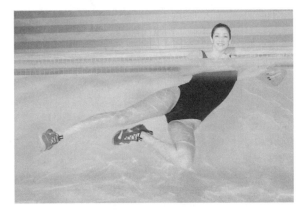

NOODLE RING

Muscle Focus: This aerobic move also works the muscles of your torso. It strengthens your torso and can help alleviate and prevent back pain.

Starting Position: Place the noodle behind your upper back and under your arms; your arms should be outstretched to either side at shoulder height and resting on the noodle. Hold your body in a straight line from your head to your toe; keep your chest lifted and a rock belly, with neutral pelvic posture. For added stability and slightly increased resistance, grasp a second noodle held horizontally in front with both hands.

Action:

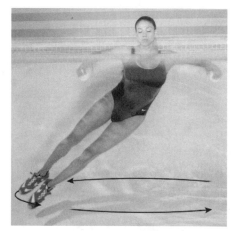

1. This move requires you to use your torso as your means of locomotion, forming a "funnel cone" that looks somewhat like a slow-moving, upside-down tornado. Alternately contract your trunk muscles on the right, front, left, and back in order to trace a large, counterclockwise circle with your feet. You will spin in a clockwise direction because, as Newton said, "for every action, there is an equal and opposite reaction." Continue for 10 to 20 seconds.

2. Repeat in the opposite direction, moving the whole body so that your feet circle in a clockwise circle: left, front, right, and back. You will spin in a counterclockwise motion as you make a funnel cone circling clockwise.

Variation: Noodle Twist

Perform in the same manner as the Noodle Ring, except with your heels together and your knees out to either side. This move opens up your spine to release tension and works the oblique muscles of the abdomen and the sides.

Safety Tip: Keep shoulder blades back and down. Don't allow your shoulders to ride up toward your ears. Use firm abdominals to protect your back.

Kickboard Moves

Incorporate the kickboard to add new challenges and whimsy to your workout with very little monetary investment. The buoyancy of the board creates a challenge to strength, balance, coordination, and stabilization.

KICKBOARD CLIMB

Purpose: This move works your lower body aerobically. It strengthens and tones your abdominals and legs: It works your abdominals and your upper-body stabilizers in an isometric contraction and challenges balance and coordination.

Starting Position: Move to the pool wall in chest-deep water, holding onto the kickboard with both hands. Adopt the position of the Plank—with your body and legs in a straight line.

Action: Contract your abdominal muscles firmly. Maintain a firm contraction throughout the exercise.

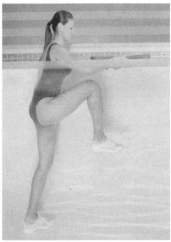

1. Powerfully raise your right knee while keeping your left foot on the floor.
2. Push off with your left leg and switch the position of your legs.
3. Continue hopping, while switching legs with a pumping action, for 8 to 32 repetitions.

Variation: Increase the challenge by moving your body at a 45-degree angle with the pool floor.

Safety Tips: Keep your knees slightly bent and your abdominals pulled in firmly. Avoid this exercise if you have neck pain.

Purpose: This move is for having fun moving about the pool and using your upper and lower body aerobically while you challenge your balance and coordination.

Starting position: Sitting on a kickboard, keep your balance by using your torso stabilizer muscles.

Action:

1. Kick your legs alternately in a flexion and extension pattern.
2. Scoop the water back in a breaststroke or sculling motion (push the water back as you move your arms along your sides, pick them up, and scoop again, like rowing) (figures *a*, *b*).
3. To increase intensity, use your arm and leg movements to move about the pool, covering distance as quickly as you can.

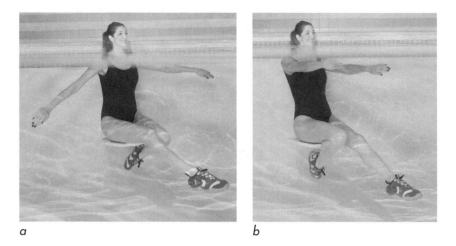

a   *b*

Safety Tip: Use your abdominals and stabilizer muscles in your sides and back to stay in an upright position rather than letting your spine curve into a C shape.

Water Country Line Dancing

Saddle up with your favorite country music and awaken your country-loving senses with water line dancing. Build on these moves by adding any of your favorite line dance steps; slow down the tempo to allow for the greater viscosity of water compared to land-based dancing. Take half the number of steps per musical stanza; that is, move half-fast!

Purpose

Insert these aerobic country line dancing moves into your aerobic warm-up and cool-down sections to put some Southern sizzle into your steps and to challenge your balance and coordination.

Starting Position

All of the steps begin with your feet a comfortable distance apart; stand upright in the braced neutral position.

Safety and Technique Tips

For all country line dancing steps, be sure to maintain healthy upright posture, with your chest open, your shoulder blades back and down, your abdominals contracted, your spine in neutral position (neither tipped forward nor back: the braced neutral posture). Move from your hips and use your buttocks and thighs as your prime movers. Move your arms to positions that allow you to maintain your balance, or tuck your thumbs into your waistband to create more surface area and challenge your balance. Maintain a speed in water that is slower than if you were dancing on land.

Water Country Line Dancing Sequence

To make the whole workout into a line dancing session, start with some light "two step" water walking in a circular or snake pattern (meaning step quick-quick, slow; quick-quick, slow), complete a stretch sequence before the dance steps, add some hops and Knee Lifts to your line dance moves, and follow the line dancing with a cool-down and stretch series.

ROCK STEP

Starting Position: Put your right foot in front and your left foot back, about half your foot's length apart between your right heel and the toes of your left foot (figure a).

Action:

1. Rock steps are similar to the Rocking Horse, but you use little steps, small enough to change slightly where you put your weight: on your front or back foot.
2. Rock forward on your right (shift your weight onto your right foot).
3. Step back onto your left (shift your weight backward onto your left foot).
4. Repeat 8 to 32 times.
5. Change to a starting position with your left foot front and your right foot back. Repeat 8 to 32 times.

Variation: Cross Rocks

Cross your right foot over your left foot: Step with your right foot in front and to the left of your left little (pinky) toe (your weight goes to the right) (figure b). Rock Step in place (shift your weight backward onto your left foot). Shift your weight forward onto your right foot. Repeat, rocking forward and back, 8 to 32 times. Cross your left foot over your right foot and repeat the forward and back rocking motion 8 to 32 times. To increase intensity, add a Knee Lift or a hop after you cross over in front.

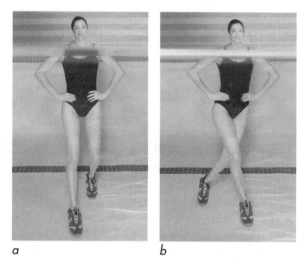

a b

SAILOR JAZZ STEP

Action:

1. Moving to the left, cross your right foot behind your left leg (figure a).
2. Step with your left foot to your left side (figure b).
3. Step with your right foot to your right and slightly forward; your weight goes to the right (figure c).
4. The move follows this sequence: Step behind, step side, step side.
5. Perform the sequence again on the opposite side, while you are moving to the right.
6. Repeat 8 to 32 times.

Variation: For heightened intensity, lift your right knee at the end of Sailor Jazz Step to the right and your left knee at the end of Sailor Jazz Step to the left.

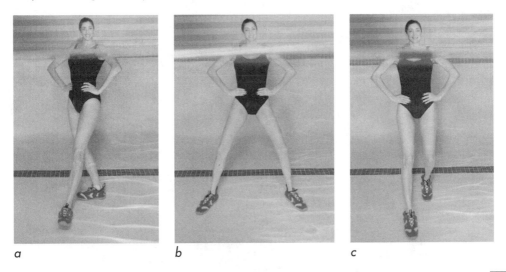

a b c

STEP-TOGETHER

Action:

1. Move to the right: Step about a shoulder width to the right and then bring your left foot next to your right foot (figures *a*, *b*). Hook your thumbs into your waistband or add some cowboy or cowgirl arm movements for fun.

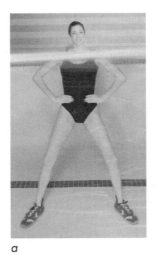 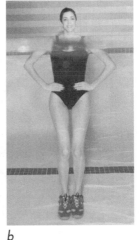

a b

2. Move to the left: Step about a shoulder width to the left and then bring your right foot next to your left foot.

3. Repeat 8 to 32 times.

Variation: Step-Together-Step

Move to the right: Step with your right foot to the right side (about a foot wide). Your weight is on your right foot. Move your left foot to the right, to bring your feet together (your weight goes to the left). Step with your right foot to the right (your weight goes to the right). Move to the left: Step with your left foot to the left side (about a foot wide); your weight is on the left. Step with your right foot next to your left, to bring your feet together; your weight goes to the right. Step with your left foot to the left (your weight goes to the left). Repeat 8 to 32 times. To increase intensity, turn the side step into a side hop.

COWBOY HIP-HOP: STEP AND STOMP

Action:

1. Step forward with your right foot (figure *a*).
2. With your left foot, take a gigantic step to the left and bring your feet together (figure *b*).
3. With your right foot, step to the left, behind your left leg (figure *c*).
4. With your left foot, step to the left.
5. Stomp together with your right foot (add a hop for more impact) (figure *d*).
6. Repeat 8 to 16 times.
7. Perform the same sequence, starting with your left foot, and repeat 8 to 16 times.

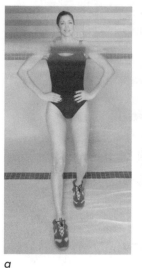

a

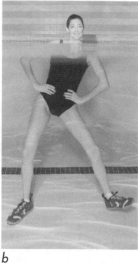

b

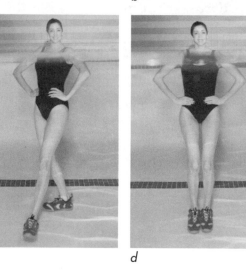

c   *d*

HONKY-TONK KICK: RIGHT AND LEFT KICK CROSS

Action:

1. Kick your right foot out to the right side (figure *a*).
2. Cross your right foot behind your left foot (figure *b*).
3. Kick your left foot out to the left side.
4. Cross left foot in front of right.

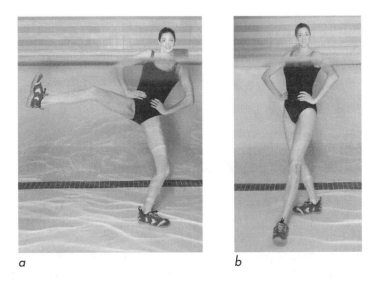

a   b

Variation: For greater intensity, add a hop as you cross your foot in front and kick the opposite leg out to the side.

Water Tai Chi

Tai Chi is based on the laws of nature. Movements and postures relate to the animals, sea, sky, and waterways of Earth. The rounded, flowing, and fluid movements lend themselves beautifully to adaptations created especially for the water: The graceful moves unique to this ancient martial art blend in a complementary way with the resistant yet relaxing qualities of movement in water.

Purpose

Water Tai Chi connects the mind and body in an aquatic environment with practices that increase vitality and energy and recharge the spirit. It delivers benefits that build on the qualities of water exercise by enhancing balance, agility, strength, flexibility, grace, coordination, posture, and mental focus. The results are increased energy and an enhanced sense of well-being, relaxation, and tranquility.

The slow movements of Tai Chi, an ancient Chinese self-defense form, move your body and mind through developments that bring spiritual growth. The definition of Tai Chi is "supreme ultimate," and the word "Chi" translates as "energy." Chi is the energy that flows through the 14 meridians of your body. These mind-body-spirit paths are like the waterways of the Earth: When the waterways are open, water flows freely. Strength and vitality arise from the flow of Chi, or universal life energy that can empower you to find balance and energy from within.

Basic Principles

The Yang style consists of a series of 100 continuous movements or postures. The movements we have selected are moves that introduce the beauty of Tai Chi in water. Yang style develops softness and strength simultaneously.

Safety and Technique Tips

Yin and Yang, the basic elements of Tai Chi, can be described as calm and active energy. Chi flows only when these two forces are in balance. In many Tai Chi postures, your feet are firmly grounded on the Earth while your upper body remains free and airy. In this way, Tai Chi forms move your body through a free-flowing, centered discipline that is rooted in the Earth by the planting of your feet, is issued through your legs, derives its control from your hips, pelvis, and waist (your body's center), and is fluidly expressed with your hands.

To keep the energy pathways open, keep your back straight and your head held erect as if it were suspended from above. Your breathing is deep and relaxed, yet your mind is alert and focused. Movement and energy originate from the center of your body, and your hand positions are graceful and expressive. Keep the joints of your arms relaxed, with your shoulders and elbows down, releasing all of the tension and tightness in your neck and shoulders. To understand the fluidity of the movement, imagine moving your arms as if they were water flowing gently. Think of your body as one of many graceful linkages and then coordinate the movements like a string of pearls.

The speed of Tai Chi movement in water is faster than on land. This difference allows you to maintain a comfortable body temperature despite the warmth-wicking environment of the water. Move to a water depth that is between the middle of your rib cage and your chest to ensure good footing and stabilization of your feet. For Tai Chi, the root is in your feet: Aquatic shoes protect your feet as well as improve your grounding and stabilization.

Water Tai Chi Sequence

Perform a Tai Chi sequence using the following moves or insert the moves into your water workout during warm-up and cool-down for added variety and serenity.

CIRCLE THE DRUM

Starting Position: Stand with your right foot in front of your left foot, at a comfortable distance from front to back that provides good stability.

Action: The basic action is ward off and pull back.

1. Roll back to shift your weight to your back leg.
2. Shift your weight to your front leg and move your hands as if you were circling a large base drum, held at your torso, as you would in a marching band. Make two large parallel circles, side by side, moving forward, away from your body, down, back toward your body again (figures a-c), and then up and circling down again.
3. When pressing forward, press your palms forward, away from your body: This is the empty (Yin) aspect of the move. When pulling back, turn the palms toward your body: This is the full (Yang) aspect of the move.
4. Transfer your weight from your front leg to your back leg as your hands move backward.
5. Transfer your weight from your back leg to your front leg as your hands move forward.
6. Pivot turn on your feet and perform the movements with your left leg in front.
7. Maintain a softness of movement with your hands and arms.
8. Repeat 8 to 16 times.

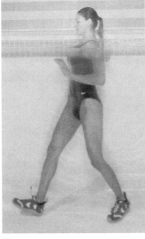
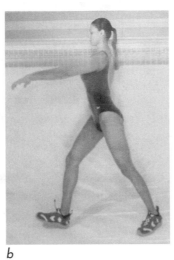
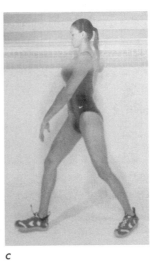

a   b   c

EMBRACING THE MOON

Starting Position: Make a transition so that you can place your feet a comfortable distance apart from left to right.

Action:

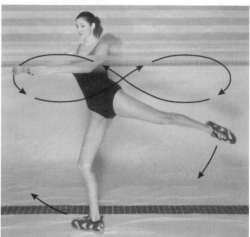

1. Visualize gently "holding" a ball of Chi energy between your hands, about 6 inches (15 cm) in diameter. Make a figure eight horizontally, from left to right, using the motion of your torso and arms.

2. Add Side Leg Lifts: Begin lifting the leg on the side opposite of your hands.

3. Repeat 8 to 16 times.

KICK BACK AND FRONT

Starting Position: Stand on one leg.

Action:

1. Kick forward and backward without touching down your foot (figures *a*, *b*).

2. Hold your fist loosely, not clenched (your fingertips gently touch the center of your palm) with each hand. Hold your thumb lightly over your fingers, with your palms down. Hold your arms out to the sides.

3. Pivot on your standing foot and make quarter turns to kick in all four directions.

4. Keep your abdominals and buttocks contracted in the braced neutral position.

5. Repeat 8 to 16 times.

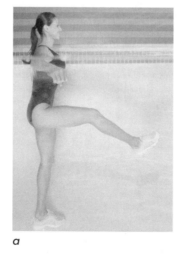

a

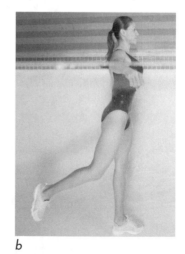

b

ARM CIRCLING

Starting Position: Spread your feet apart from left to right.

Action:

1. Fluidly move your arm across the front of your chest as if you were smoothing the air at chest level, and then draw back across your chest and out to the side, forming a wide oval: Reach out, across, pull back, and out, reaching slightly behind. Your torso turns slightly with your arm movements (figures a, b).

2. Shift your weight from one leg to the other in the same direction as your arms.

3. Complete 8 repetitions; repeat with the opposite side.

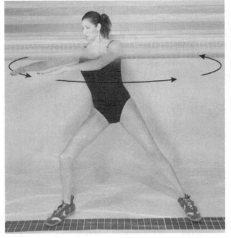 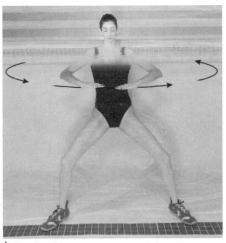

a   b

SCOOP THE EARTH

Starting Position: Adopt a Forward Lunge position, with your front knee bent, while resting on the balls of your feet (figure *a*).

Action:

1. Float your arms to the surface of the water.
2. Scoop down under the water to collect the Earth's energy (full) (figure *b*), and then lift your arms up and out to the sides, letting the energy flow through your arms and out through your fingertips (empty) as you shift your weight back (figure *c*).
3. Pivot turn on the balls of your feet, with your arms lifted out to the sides, so that you are lunging in the opposite direction. Repeat on the other side.
4. Alternate for 8 to 32 repetitions.

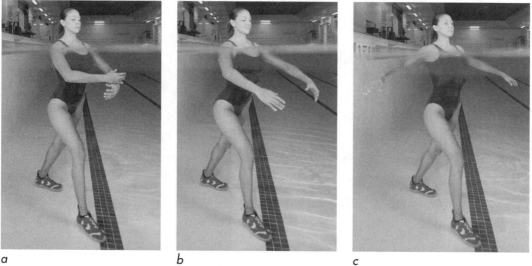

a   b   c

PAT HIGH ON HORSE: PAT AND PULL

Starting Position: Adopt the Forward Lunge position, with your left foot forward, your front knee bent, your right foot back and turned slightly out. Bend your elbows, with your hands in ready position in front of your chest.

Action:

1. Turn your left palm forward and your right palm backward (figure *a*). Push your left palm forward and pull your right palm backward. Watch the hand moving forward.
2. Turn your palms, and face your right palm forward and your left palm backward (figure *b*). Then push your right palm forward and pull your left palm backward.

3. Push your hands along the centerline of your body, keeping your elbows slightly bent and your shoulders relaxed. Maintain a soft expression in your hands.

4. Repeat 8 to 16 times.

5. Pivot turn to perform the move with your right leg in front.

6. To add the lower-body movements, start by pushing forward with your left palm and shifting your weight forward onto your left leg.

7. As you move your left hand backward, shift your weight back onto your right leg.

8. Pivot turn and, as you push forward with your right palm, shift your weight forward onto your right leg.

9. As you move your right hand backward, shift your weight back onto your left leg.

10. Repeat 8 to 16 times.

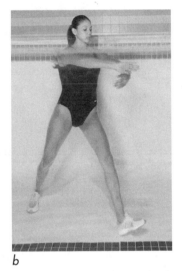

a   b

Variations:

- Vary the hand and arm position. Bring your elbows down and turn your hands so your fingertips point up.

- Combine with forward and backward striding.

- Combine Crouching Step with High Pat on Horse: Crouch down slightly and step forward and back, pivot turning on your feet to turn your hips with each step. Add the movement of your hand pushing forward and then pulling back.

MOVE 88 PARTING THE WILD HORSE'S MANE

Starting Position: Adopt the Forward Lunge position, with your left foot forward, your left knee bent, and your right foot back and turned slightly out.

Action:
1. Hold your arms as if you were cradling a child to the side (figure a).
2. Turn your front palm up and your back palm down; bring one hand forward and the other backward (figure b). Shift your weight to your back leg.
3. Return to the cradled child position and shift your weight to your front leg.
4. Pivot and repeat.
5. Repeat 8 to 16 times.

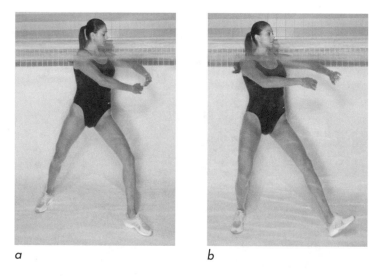

a   b

Variation: Descend into a partial squat and add a crouching step with each repetition.

Many of these water-adapted Tai Chi-style movements, inspired by water exercise adaptations by Carol Argo of the Aquatic Exercise Association, are included by special permission. To order a copy of the DVD *Water Tai Chi with Carol Argo: A Graceful, Flowing Shallow Water Workout,* call 1-888-544-0547 or go to www.CarolArgo.com.

Water Kickboxing

Water Kickboxing offers a fun way to release tension and pent-up stress while getting in shape. Each kickboxing move strengthens your core as well as your upper- and lower-body muscles in an integrated fashion. According to the International Fitness Association, kickboxing follows these basic guidelines.

Purpose

Water kickboxing develops overall strength and agility conditioning and muscle toning, and releases stress.

Starting Position

All kickboxing moves begin with this starting position. Perform these moves in chest-deep water. Keep your body in a neutral position—neither arch nor round your back. Keep your abdominal muscles tight. Stand with your feet shoulder-width apart. For greater stability, perform these moves in a forward lunge position.

Safety and Technique Tips

- Never lock out your knees and elbows (keep them "soft").
- Keep your body in a neutral position—neither arch nor round your back.
- Always keep your abdominal muscles tight.
- All kicks should be low kicks.
- The music should be at about 122 to 128 beats per minute so that you can complete each move with proper form. (Slower in water.)
- While you are doing high impact footwork, keep light on the balls of your feet. Imagine that you're on a glass floor.
- Make your whole leg act as a shock absorber.

Kickboxing Sequence

Insert these moves into your overall water workout as a transition following your aerobic section or as part of your strengthening and toning exercises.

FORWARD JAB

MOVE
89

Action:

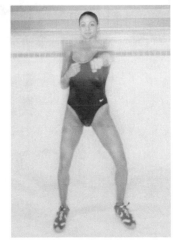

1. Punch with your first two knuckles, using the flat part.
2. Keep your elbow tucked in close to your body to avoid irritation of your rotator cuff and deltoid (shoulder) muscles. Keeping your elbow close to your body also adds power to the punch.
3. Maintain a straight alignment from your hand to your shoulder.
4. Repeat 8 to 16 times.

Safety Tips: Maintain balance. Keep your shoulder blades down and avoid artificially raising your shoulder; allow only a slight rise in your shoulder.

CROSS JAB

Action:

1. This move is the same as the Forward Jab except that it crosses the centerline of your body.
2. Twist your left hip forward.
3. As you punch forward with your right fist, rotate your torso into the punch.
4. Push off the ground with the heel of your foot.
5. Repeat 8 to 16 times.

Safety Tip: Maintain your knee and toe in alignment to prevent your knee from twisting or torquing (moving with a twisting force). Your knee should point in the same direction as your first and second toes.

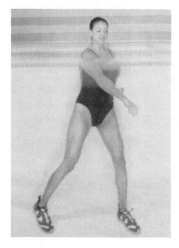

SHIN BLOCK

Action:

1. Raise your knee to your chest (figure *a*).
2. Bring your opposite shoulder in slightly, similar to a Standing Crunch (figure *b*).
3. Return your leg to the starting position.
4. Repeat 8 to 16 times.

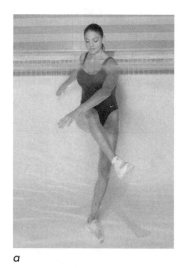
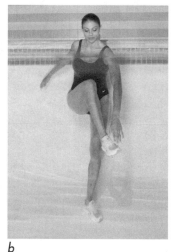

a   *b*

KNEE STRIKE

Action:

1. Raise your knee to your chest (figure *a*).
2. Reach up with both hands and pull the (visualized) target down onto your knee.
3. Return your leg to the starting position (figure *b*).
4. Repeat 8 to 16 times.

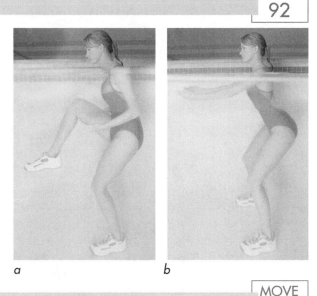

a   b

FRONT KICK FROM REAR LEG OR FRONT LEG

Action:

1. Initiate the Front Kick by bringing your knee up first (figure *a*).
2. Point your knee at the target and then kick. Extend (kick out) your lower leg. Avoid snapping or hyperextending your knee (figure *b*).
3. Bring your leg down to the original position with control and maintain balance.
4. Repeat 8 to 16 times.

Variation: Turning Kick

Adopt a Side Fighting Stance, in a defense position, with one foot forward. The Turning Kick is similar to the Front Kick except for a slight turn into the kick. Transfer your weight to the ball of your rear foot, then raise your knee toward the target and begin the extension of your knee and contact the (visualized) target with the top of your foot. Bring your leg down to the starting position. Repeat 8 to 16 times.

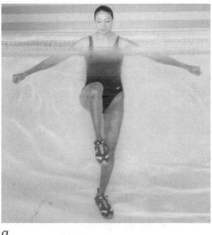 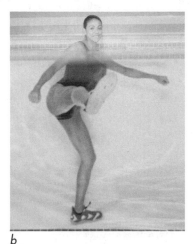

a   b

Water Yoga

The fluid movements of yoga adapt naturally to the aquatic environment. Practice in the yoga tradition, with a focus on breathing and a light, loving heart.

Purpose

Water yoga techniques enhance flexibility, balance, and strength in a soothing series of moves that calm your mind. With regular practice, the mind-body-spirit integration of water yoga can bring you relaxation, improved posture and breathing, and an enhanced sense of body awareness.

Safety and Technique Tips

Perform these movements in water at the depth of the middle of your rib cage or in more shallow water if you have trouble keeping your feet in contact with the floor. Wear aqua shoes to gain greater control and stability. Keep your breathing active, inhaling and exhaling through your nose. Deep breathing is central to yoga practice.

All yoga moves and positions require maintaining a strong core by bracing your body in neutral position, with your back neither arched nor rounded.

Water Yoga Sequence

First, warm up with water walking by using gradually lengthening forward and back strides, followed by side steps. Follow with these yoga poses and movements that have been specially modified to work well in the water. End with stretches that cool your torso, legs, and arms in a relaxed, lengthened position (Stretches #1 through 19).

MOVE 94 | SALUTATION TO THE SUN

Purpose: Traditionally, the Salutation to the Sun communicates that the divine light in each of us honors the divine light in you. This move can warm up your body as if you were standing in the rays of the sun and enhance your range of motion. It opens your mind, body, and spiritual awareness to the universe.

Starting Position: Perform this exercise in chest- to shoulder-deep water. Stand with one foot in front of the other at a comfortable distance apart that provides good stability. Contract your abdominal and buttocks muscles to brace your spine in neutral position. Keep your chest lifted and your shoulder blades down and back. Your shoulders should be partly submerged.

Action:

1. Contract your abdominal muscles to keep your lower back from arching.
2. Press one leg behind you as you bend your front knee as in a lunge, and bring both arms overhead.
3. Hold the pose for several seconds.
4. Bring your arms down.
5. Step together.
6. Repeat with your other leg.
7. Repeat the sequence for 8 to 16 repetitions.

Safety Tip: Make a particular effort to keep your shoulder blades squeezed together and down.

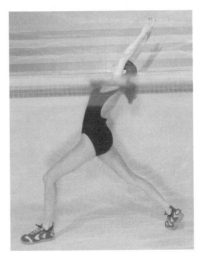

BOW AND ARROW IN WARRIOR POSE

Purpose: The Warrior Pose teaches you how to bring wisdom, courage, and unwavering focus into the actions of your everyday life. It is a powerful pose, but, as you explore the alignment and inner attitude of the pose, the heart of the peaceful warrior begins to reveal itself. Like a Zen archer focusing on a bull's-eye—who practices just holding a bow for two years before ever releasing an arrow—find balance within your focus by becoming inwardly observant and calm. Enhance the integrated strength and range of motion in your chest, your upper back, your middle and lower torso, and your hips and buttocks.

Starting Position: Stand with your legs wide apart and your right knee bent. Align your front knee directly over your ankle. Turn your back foot out. The heel of your front leg is in a straight line with the arch of your back foot.

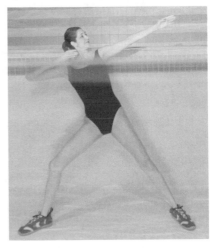

Action:

1. Reach straight out with your left arm.
2. Reach your right hand toward your left hand and then pull back as if you are drawing an arrow back against a bowstring.
3. Repeat the sequence for 8 to 16 repetitions.

FLAMINGO OR SUPERMAN POSE

Purpose: In this pose, balance like a flamingo on one leg. The move can relax your mind and body, improve your core strength, and enhance your musculo-skeletal alignment.

Action:

1. Raise one straight leg up behind you, with your arms out to the sides and slightly back. Form the shape of Superman flying, but with one leg down and with your arms out to your sides at shoulder level.
2. Drop your chin to lengthen the back of your neck (figure a).
3. Hold the pose for 10 to 20 seconds on each leg.

Variation: Warrior Three pose: Raise both arms in front of you (figure b).

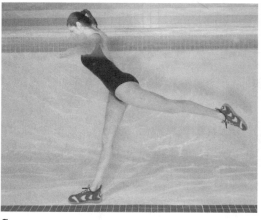 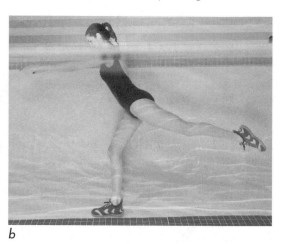

a   b

HALF LOTUS

Purpose: The Indian Lotus flower symbolizes divinity, fertility, wealth, knowledge, and enlightenment. The Half Lotus is named so because the position puts the soles of your feet up, reminiscent of a lotus flower. The move stretches your deep buttocks muscles and relaxes pent-up tension. The Half Lotus is similar to Stretch #10, Deep-Muscle Hip, Thigh, and Buttocks Stretch.

Starting Position: Face the pool wall, with both hands on the edge.

Action:

1. Cross your right ankle just above your left knee and slowly lower yourself as if you were sitting in a chair. Keep your back straight and press your hips way back (figure a).
2. Relax your buttocks, hip, and outer thigh; contract your abdominal muscles; breathe deeply. Hold for 10 to 20 seconds.

3. Reach out to the sides and then scull (glide your hands through the water with cupped palms): Move your arms forward and backward, just under the surface of the water, to maintain balance and keep your body warm (figure b).

4. Put both feet on the floor and stand up; then repeat with your left ankle at your right knee.

5. Hold the position for 10 to 20 seconds on each side.

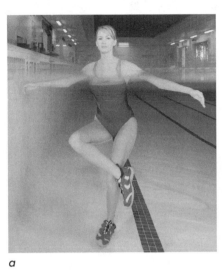
a

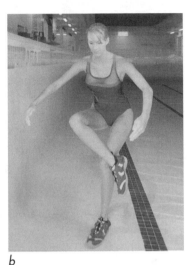
b

HALF MOON

Purpose: This move radiates quiet strength, like the light of the moon. Strong engagement of your entire body makes this pose invigorating and effective for strength and poise.

Action:

1. Lift one leg out to the side, with the opposite arm down and the same arm up. Radiate strength from your center. Extend your body out to imitate the shape of a starfish.

2. Move slowly from one leg to the other, projecting strong lines of energy out of your body.

3. After several repetitions, hold the position for several seconds on each side.

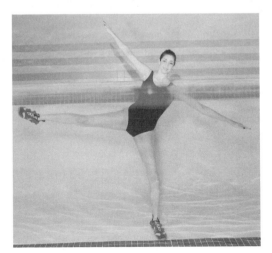

TREE POSE

Purpose: The tree symbolizes growth with your roots connected to the Earth. It improves balance and quiets tension in your muscles. The Tree Pose creates the feeling of being centered and focused with a sense of firm foundation.

Action:

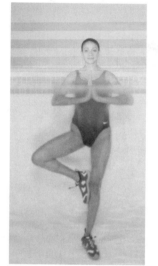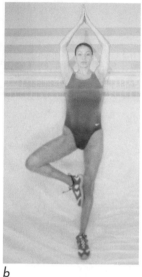

1. Place the sole of your foot on the inside of your thigh or lower leg.

2. Place your palms together at your breastbone, with your fingers pointing up. Press your elbows out to the sides (figure *a*).

3. Sweep your arms apart and overhead; lift and raise them to the sky. Your palms meet overhead, with your elbows bent (figure *b*).

a   *b*

4. Softly bring your arms back down.

5. Hold the pose for 10 to 20 seconds.

Variation: Move to the wall for added stability. Turn your back to the wall and place the heel of your supporting leg against the wall.

TRIANGLE EXTENDED SIDE-ANGLE POSE

Purpose: This move demonstrates the yoga principle called active alignment; it helps center your posture and your mind. It strengthens and stretches your ankles, knees, groin, and hamstrings; it opens your chest and shoulders, improves circulation to the muscles around your spine, and stimulates your organs.

Action:

1. Inhale deeply; on exhalation, step or lightly jump, with your feet 3.5 to 4 feet (1 to 1.2 m) apart. Raise your arms parallel to the floor and reach them actively out to your sides, with your palms down and your chest open.

2. Turn your left foot slightly to the right, and turn your right foot out 90 degrees. Align your left heel with your right heel. Contract your thigh muscles, and turn your right thigh outward. Bend your right knee and position your feet far enough apart so that your knee is directly in line over the center of your left ankle. Inhale.

3. Exhale; extend your torso to the right, directly over your right leg, bending from your hip joint, not your waist. Anchor this movement by engaging

the muscles of your left leg and pressing your outer heel firmly to the floor. Rotate your torso to the left. Let your left hip come slightly forward and lengthen your tailbone toward your back heel.

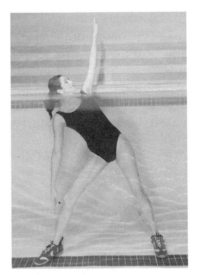

4. Rest your right hand on your shin or on your thigh just above your knee, whatever is possible without distorting the aligned positioning at the sides of your torso. Stretch your left arm toward the sky, in line with the tops of your shoulders, creating a diagonal line. Keep your head and neck in a neutral position or turn it to the right, with your eyes gazing softly at your left thumb.

5. Stay in this pose for 10 to 30 seconds to 1 minute. Inhale to come up, strongly pressing your back heel into the floor and reaching your top arm toward the ceiling.

6. Reverse your feet; change sides and repeat the pose for the same length of time to the right.

7. Feel your entire body engaged in the movement and stretch.

Many of these water-adapted movements inspired by Hatha yoga are included by special permission from Carol Argo of the Aquatic Exercise Association. The DVD, *Water Yoga with Carol Argo, Stretch, Strengthen, & Center the Mind and Body*, provides a full yoga workout adapted to the water. To order the DVD, call 1-888-544-0547 or go to www.CarolArgo.com.

Water Pilates

Insert Water Pilates into your strengthening and toning section, or make your whole session a Water Pilates Workout by warming up gently, performing a thorough stretch sequence, completing each of the Water Pilates moves, and then finishing with a comprehensive cool-down stretch sequence.

Purpose

Pilates trains your body to move as an integrated whole. The methods focus on enhanced body awareness, energy, posture, and breathing. Pilates builds a stronger core by working from your body's center and outward. Performing Water Pilates moves can help you develop and maintain strong, flexible function and an elongated body, results that are beneficial for all ages and fitness levels.

The advantage of Pilates is that it trains your body in a manner consistent with the enhanced strength and flexibility needed for how you use your body in day-to-day life and in recreational or sport activities. The focus is on the muscles that stabilize your spine and joints; the movement challenges that stabilization in order to build strength and stability.

Safety and Technique Tips

For each of the moves, begin by standing in shallow water, chest to shoulder depth. Lengthen your spine upward, draw your shoulders down, and contract your abdominal muscles. Concentrate on stabilization first, movement second. After you have mastered these moves and begin to feel only moderately challenged, add resistance equipment for your lower body, your upper body, or both, in order to expand the challenge. Be sure that your stabilizer muscles are truly up to the task or you risk injury.

If you take a break from Water Pilates for a few days or weeks, start back at a lower level of challenge, generally without equipment. Pilates techniques can be extremely effective within a shorter time frame than some other techniques. Because of the intensive effects of Pilates, proper form and training techniques—such as adhering to the principle of returning to workouts at a lesser intensity when training has ceased for any elapsed time—become even more crucial and imperative.

During each exercise, focus on proper body alignment and full breathing, drawing your breath deeply into your abdomen as opposed to shallow breathing into your chest cavity alone.

Water Pilates Sequence

A Pilates sequence begins with a warm-up consisting of an easy jog, side steps, Pomp and Circumstance, Knee Lifts, lunges, and movements that combine these exercises. Use nonbounding moves for the warm-up: Pilates involves slow and steady motion. Follow the warm-up with a thorough stretch sequence, concentrating mostly on your lower body.

MOVE 101   SAW

Muscle Focus: This move targets your hip, pelvic, buttocks, oblique abdominals, and hamstring muscles via rotation of your hip and torso.

Starting Position: Position your legs in a wide stance, left to right, and bring your arms out to the sides.

Action:

1. Squat with both arms out to the sides, with your palms down.
2. Slowly twist to the right while looking at the arm reaching behind your body; hold the position (figure a). Inhale and exhale deeply.
3. Again, slowly twist to the left and hold the position while looking at your back arm.

4. External rotation: Lift the left leg (slightly bent) out to the side while rotating your hip outward. Simultaneously turn your torso toward your lifted leg and reach your right arm toward your opposite foot (figure *b*). Reach your little finger toward your little toe. Repeat 8 to 32 times with your left leg and then with your right leg, or alternate legs.

5. Internal Rotation: Kick out in front diagonally, across your body, while reaching your opposite hand toward your toes (figure *c*). Bring your leg back to the starting position and repeat. Repeat 8 to 32 times with your left leg and then with your right leg.

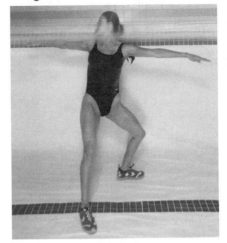

a

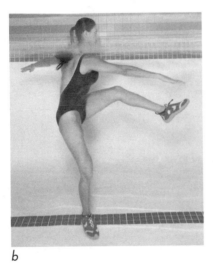

b

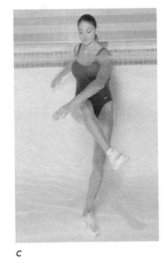

c

Variation: When you slowly twist, instead of keeping your back arm straight out, bend your elbow so that your arms are in a bow and arrow position.

Safety Tips: Hinge from your hip; keep your spine long and your torso upright and avoid collapsing at your rib cage. End with a rotational range of motion and stretch. When stretching, move through your comfortable range of motion with easy rotation at the waist, gliding slowly from left to right and right to left, with your arms outstretched. Reach around your body, with one forearm resting on the front of your body at your waist and one arm in back. Stretch and hold the position. Switch arms and repeat.

HALF-MOON TIGHTROPE TOUCH

Muscle Focus: This move enhances posture by strengthening your core. It works the muscles of your hips, buttocks, and thighs.

Starting Position: Imagine that you are standing on a tightrope, with your right leg in front and your arms out to the sides just below the surface of the water (figure a).

Action:

1. Stabilize your core and use the muscles of your pelvis, waist, hips, and buttocks to change the position of your leg: With a straight leg, touch the tightrope in front with your toes.

2. Sweep your leg out to the side and back, with your toe tracing the form of a half circle, and touch the tightrope behind you (figures b, c).

3. Sweep your leg forward, tracing a half circle, to touch the tightrope in front of you again.

4. Repeat 8 to 16 times, first with your right leg and then with your left leg.

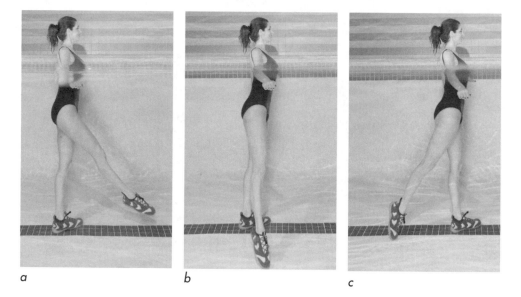

a   b   c

Variation: Add torso rotation: As you touch forward, gently turn your torso toward the opposite leg in front and then away from your leg in back. As you bring your left leg forward, rotate your right side toward your left leg, with your arms outstretched at the surface of the water.

Safety Tips: Stretch your leg out long, from the hip. Lengthen your spine, engage your abdominal muscles, and keep your shoulder blades down and back. Keep your pelvis in a neutral position, with a firm, rock belly, using your stabilizer muscles. Movement radiates out from your center. Elongate your body during all movement. Move smoothly, fluidly, and gracefully. After completing this exercise, step wide apart and release your back by an easy torso rotation, with your arms out to the sides.

LEG CIRCLES

Muscle Focus: This move works the muscles of your hips, thighs, and buttocks and challenges the stabilizers of your torso.

Starting Position: Stand by the wall. With one arm, hold the wall for stability; reach your other arm out toward the middle of the pool.

Action:

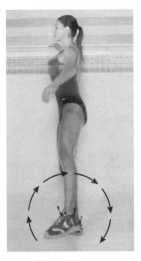

1. Lift one leg out to the side to make large circles. Keep your torso upright and your pelvis braced in a neutral position.
2. Point your toe for maximum stretch and to lengthen the lever for increased resistance.
3. Repeat 8 to 16 times in each direction. Turn around and repeat equally on the opposite side.

Variations:

- Move your extended arm forward and back.
- Vary the circle size. Use small circles and imagine you are circling your leg inside a small hoop.
- Slip a swim noodle behind your back, outstretch your arms to either side and wrap them around the noodle. Contract your abdominal muscles and lift your legs out in front, keeping them relatively straight. Form circles of varying sizes with both legs simultaneously. Repeat 8 to 32 times.

Safety Tips: Engage your buttocks and abdominal muscles. Extend your torso upward to open up your spine. In Pilates, much of the work is done in the stabilization. To modify, reduce the range of motion by making smaller circles. Make the action of the circles originate from the top of your leg and your hip joint.

DIAGONAL BICYCLE PUMP

Muscle Focus: This move works the muscles of your hips, thighs, and buttocks and challenges the stabilizers of your torso.

Starting Position: Stand by the wall. With one arm, hold the wall for stability; reach your other arm out toward the middle of the pool. Challenge your stabilizer muscles by performing this move in the diagonal position to increase torso fitness while working your legs, hips, and buttocks. In other words, tilt your body on a diagonal. Hold on to the wall with one hand, and step both feet away from the wall, several steps out to the side. Keep your whole torso taut and in line with your legs, forming a straight diagonal line from your head to your toe. Support your weight on the poolside arm, and reach out toward the middle of the pool with the opposite arm. Rest your weight on the outer edge of your foot (figure a).

Action:

1. Using your outside leg, bring your knee up (figure b).
2. Extend your leg, pressing down and around as you would in pedaling a bicycle.
3. Repeat 8 to 32 times and then turn around and switch legs.

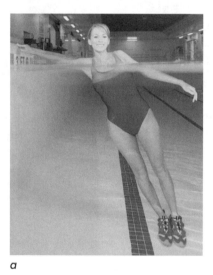
a

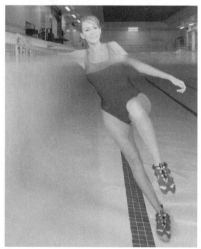
b

Variation: As you pump, press your leg down and then back behind you instead of simply straight down and as you press back, concentrate on engaging your abdominal muscles and on elongating your psoas muscle, the hip flexor muscle between your thigh and your torso.

Safety Tip: Maintain a very firm abdominal contraction to protect your back and strengthen your core.

Muscle Focus: This torso-challenging Chest Press strengthens your spine, abdominals, upper body, and pelvic stability and improves your posture.

Starting Position: Hold two swim noodles or long-handled flotation bells in both hands in front of your body, with your arms just wider than shoulder-width apart. Stabilize your body in a straight line: Keep your legs straight, brace your pelvis in neutral position, and keep your chest open and lifted. The work is in maintaining that stabilized position. Squeeze your buttocks and elongate your body upward, with your shoulder blades down and back. Lengthen your neck by lifting up through the crown of your head, opening the space between the vertebrae in your neck.

Action:

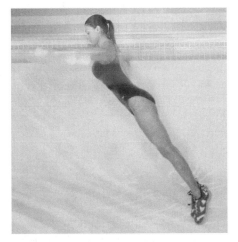

1. Move your feet backward to form a diagonal line with your body from your head to your toe, with your legs behind you and the swim noodle held in front.

2. Stabilize your torso: Contract your abdominal and buttocks muscles; bring your shoulder blades down and back. Maintain this stabilization throughout the move: This represents the torso-strengthening action of this exercise.

3. Perform a Chest Press: Press the noodle forward and then pull it back slowly.

4. The point of the exercise is to maintain stability through your spine, from your head to your tailbone, and in your legs, as you perform a Chest Press against the noodle's resistance. That works the muscles of your body's core stabilizers, which enhance your day-to-day function, as well as improve sport performance and increase your resistance to injury.

Safety Tips: Inhale as the noodle comes toward your body; exhale as you press out. This exercise requires focus and concentration: Keep your body very strong. To release back tension after this exercise, bring your buttocks back and curve your back into the shape of a "c" as you hold the noodle or flotaton bell in front. To increase the challenge safely, start with two noodles held together; then reduce to one noodle as you become stronger.

MOVE 106 | OTTER

Purpose: This joyful and playful exercise releases your spine after concentrated torso work and feels great.

Starting Position: Hold the noodle in front of you in both hands, just wider than shoulder-width apart.

Action:

1. Maintaining the hold on the noodle, extend your legs out in front.
2. Spin your upper body slowly around in a circle. Allow your torso to bend gently to enhance blood flow through the back and spine, and relax the muscles.
3. Your legs are on your left side, then behind your torso, then to your right side, as you spin your upper body clockwise very slowly (figures a-c).
4. Repeat in the opposite, counterclockwise direction.

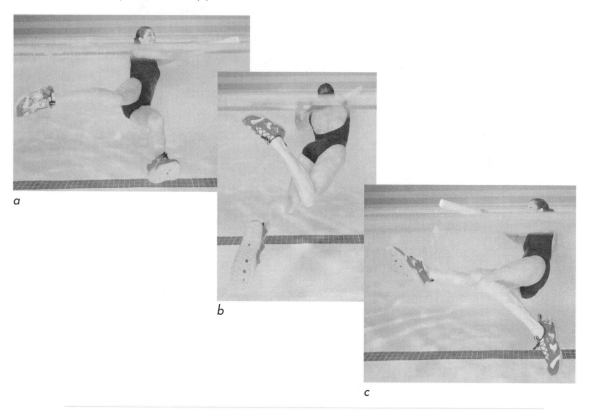

a

b

c

Yoga Booty Ballet

Yoga Booty Ballet fuses yoga, body sculpting, and dance into a fun and funky movement technique. Yoga Booty Ballet creators Gillian Marloth Clark and Teigh McDonough combined the power of quiet breathing; rejuvenation of body, mind, and spirit through yoga; concentrated body sculpting and grace-ful ballet; and the mood-lifting energy of cardio dance.

Safety and Technique Tips

The word *yoga* means to unite, and the practice of yoga brings together physi-cal postures, breathing techniques, and healing meditation. Water Yoga Booty Ballet embraces the universal yoga tradition of union, or oneness, and asks par-ticipants to begin with this mindset: I am open, I am receptive, I am worthy.

Postural techniques are central to Yoga Booty Ballet moves. Maintain a firm belly, in a braced, neutral pelvis position: Keep your tailbone down; don't arch your lower back or scoop your pelvis forward; keep your abdominal and buttocks muscles engaged. The Pelvic Scoop is a specific exercise that can be used to strengthen pelvic stabilization muscles. For instance, you perform it during squats at the top of the rise position by squeezing your abdominals and buttocks while briefly scooping your pelvis under. It also helps warm up and strengthen your pelvis stabilization muscles during Hip and Pelvic Circles, as explained later.

Get funky and use your upper-body and hip motions with "attitude" to loosen up your body, mind, and spirit. The adaptation of Yoga Booty Ballet to the aquatic environment requires that you slow down the dance movements considerably to accommodate the higher viscosity of the water.

Throughout, be sure to engage and contract the abdominal muscles in order to strengthen the body's core and protect the back. Water Yoga Booty Ballet moves require a base of core fitness; consider it advanced training.

Water Yoga Booty Ballet Sequence

The creators of land-based Yoga Booty Ballet suggest that you begin your Yoga Booty Ballet Workout with a sense of courage and willingness to aspire toward your highest potential. Set an intention at the beginning of every workout. A YBB intention that I use is, "I am present in the moment, willing to work and listening to my internal signals." Crystallize the intention before you begin, repeat it, and let it emanate from your heart and soul as you enjoy dancing the Water Yoga Booty Ballet. Finish with deep meditative breathing.

Complete a thorough thermal and stretch warm-up. Build intensity gradu-ally, and cool down gradually. Always end with relaxing stretches. Be sure to include the Full Back Stretch and Midback Stretch. Perform Yoga Booty Ballet in waist- to chest-deep water. Complete a session following the sequence listed in table 9.1, or insert the moves into your water workout according to the purpose stated for each. The workout in table 9.1 includes Water Workout moves that become Water Yoga Booty Ballet by jazzing up the action with dance, drama, or just a funky attitude. Perform Yoga Booty Ballet in waist- to chest-deep water.

These moves are inspired by Yoga Booty Ballet and appear by permission. To obtain the Yoga Booty Ballet DVDs, contact www.BeachBody.com or call 1-800-207-0420.

Table 9.1   Sample Creative Water Workout Sequence Inspired by Yoga Booty Ballet

Sequence Section	Moves	YBB Style Variation
Thermal Warm-Up and Stretch	#94 Salutation to the Sun #86 Scoop the Earth	Think about your intention and be present in the moment.
	#77 Rock Step	Funk up the move with sensual shoulder rolls or swiveling hip action (contract your abdominal muscles).
	#78 Sailor Jazz Step	Jazz it up with shoulder shimmies while holding your arms out to either side.
	#107 Stir the Pot	
	Stretches: #1-19	Move sensually through each stretch, feel the flow, and move your body through its full range of motion, especially at the hips and pelvis.
Aerobic Exercises	#108 Tailbone Swish and Swing	
	#79 Step-Together	Add shoulder shimmy, hip swivel, or double press-down with shrugs. Modulate your torso with hip action to spice up the action.
	#80 Cowboy Hip-Hop: Step and Stomp	Add some curvy hip action. Press elbows back in a pulsating rhythm.
	#81 Honky-Tonk Kick: Right and Left Kick Cross	Glide your arms across your body in opposition to the movement of the kicks.
	#16 Sailor's Jig and Knee-Lift Jig	Add a double pulsing contraction at the top of each lift.
	#109 Naughty Kitty, Good Kitty	
	#17 Jump Forward, Jump Back	Press your arms down as you jump. Use the Pelvic Scoop (see YBB move #122, Stir the Pot).
	#93 Kickboxing Variation: Turning Kick	
	#21 Knee-Lift Press-Back	1) Double the Knee Lift and change the Leg Press-Back to Rear Karate Kick with hip turn-out. 2) Double the Knee Lift and add an Oblique Abdominal Crunch at the top of the Knee Lift.

Muscle Strengthening and Toning Exercises	#96 Flamingo Pose	Add a pulsing contraction at the top of the lift (add repeated tiny lifts at lifted position).
	#102 Half-Moon Tightrope Touch	Contract the abdominals firmly and lift the leg at various points on the half moon and hold it up; at each lift, add pulsing contractions for 8 to 16 counts and then move on to the next point. Add the form and grace of ballet by using arced arm positions—overhead, in front, to the side—to balance your lifts.
	#110 Street Dance: Making Tracks	
	#34 Outer- and Inner-Thigh Scissors	Perform away from the wall. Add a double pulse (small push upward) at the top of the lift. Use your arms in opposition to the lift for balance. Keep your arms out to the sides; lift the opposite arm up overhead in a graceful balletic arc. Perform a Side Leg Lift with a hip turn-in to work your buttocks muscles.
	#54 Plank or #105 Plank and Press	
	#101 Saw	Raise your hands, with your palms up and your elbows outward at ear height, in a "Dancing Sheeba" pose.
	#61 Squat Press	Add pulsing contraction at the partial squat position. Step wider apart, turn out your toes and add hip turnout, and lift your heels. Add 8 to 16 pulsing contractions, and perform 3 sets.
	#41 Squat Touch	Perform away from the wall with arms out in front. Move into a Side Lunge and touch between squats.
	#85 Arm Circling	Deepen and raise the squat depth as you circle your arms.
	#82 Circle the Drum	Add Knee Lift and kick, alternating legs with each complete circle.
	#95 Bow and Arrow in Warrior Pose	Funk it up with double pulses on the pull-back.
Final Cool-Down Stretches	#99 Tree Pose	Relax.
	Stretches: #1–19	Move sensually through each stretch, feel the flow, and move your body through its full range of motion, especially at your hips and pelvis. Finish with deep meditative breathing.

STIR THE POT

Purpose: This move uses hip and pelvic circles to warm up your torso, pelvis, and spinal muscles.

Starting Position: Stand with your feet shoulder-width apart, with your abdominal muscles engaged to support the neutral pelvis; firm belly.

Action:

1. Circle your hips slowly clockwise with your abdominal muscles engaged. Close your hands in a loose fist, hold them near your hips, and follow the hip motion with smaller circular hand motions (figures *a*, *b*).
2. Change direction. Slowly circle your hips and hands counterclockwise.
3. Repeat 8 to 16 times in each direction.

Variation: Engage your pelvis muscles to perform Pelvic Rolls: Slowly circle your hips and pelvis, with a contraction into the "pelvic scoop" on the forward part of the circle.

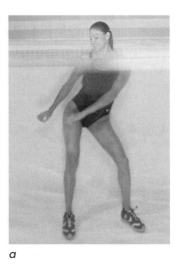 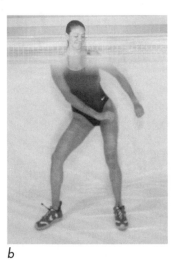

a   b

TAILBONE SWISH AND SWING

Purpose: Use this move to warm up and to loosen up and strengthen the muscles of your pelvis. It strengthens and tones your abdominal muscles.

Starting Position: Step apart and tip your hips to the right.

Action:

1. Contract your abdominal muscles and bend your elbows at your rib cage. Swish your tailbone back and forth 4 times or more. At the same time, swing your forearms back and forth from the elbow (figures *a*, *b*).

2. Tip your hips to the left and repeat the hip swish and arm swing motions.
3. Contract your abdominal muscles, jut your hip out slightly to the left and swish your tailbone back and forth 4 times or more. At the same time, put your left hand on your hip and wave your right hand in the air, front to back, from the wrist (figures c, d).
4. Tip your hips to the right and repeat the hip swish and lasso motions.

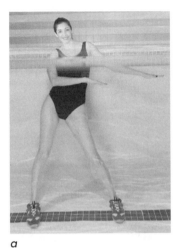

a

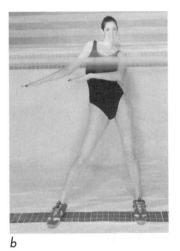

b

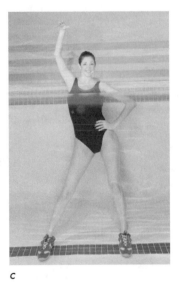

c

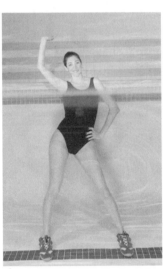

d

NAUGHTY KITTY, GOOD KITTY

Purpose: This move elevates your heart rate for aerobic conditioning; it strengthens and tones your torso.

Starting Position: Stand with your legs wide apart; turn partway to your right.

Naughty Kitty Action:

1. Swiftly step in place in a "double touch" and lunge right as you reach down across your body with your left hand (figure *a*).
2. Pull your elbow back and up to the left with a "cat's claw" dangling down, as you return to upright posture (figure *b*). Repeat 4 times.
3. Turn partway to the left and repeat the motion on the other side, reaching and pulling back with your right arm. Repeat 4 times.
4. Repeat the entire sequence 8 to 16 times, and intersperse it with other moves.

Good Kitty Action:

1. Slow down the motion. Smoothly step in place and lunge right as you contract and shorten your right oblique abdominals (the right side of your torso) while coquettishly dipping your left shoulder down (by contracting your abdominal muscles) (figure *c*). Avoid rolling your shoulder forward. Repeat 4 times.
2. Turn partway to the left and repeat the motion, contracting your left oblique abdominals while coquettishly dipping your right shoulder down. Repeat 4 times.
3. Repeat the entire sequence 8 to 16 times, and intersperse it with other moves.

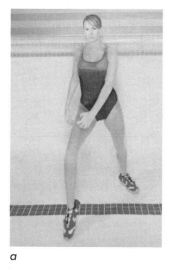

a

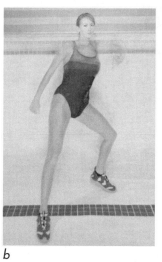

b

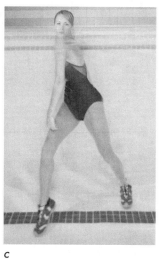

c

Purpose: This move increases your aerobic endurance, tones your legs, hips, and buttocks, and challenges your core strength.

Starting Position: Stand with your feet shoulder-width apart and imagine that you are standing with both feet just inside a set of railroad tracks. Stand upright, with your torso and back stabilized using the braced neutral position. Rock belly contractions make this move work your abdominals and strengthen your core.

Action:

1. Funk up the attitude as you imagine stepping out over the tracks.
2. Powerfully lift your right knee toward your chest as you squat and step over the right track (figure *a*).
3. Stomp your foot down outside the track (figure *b*).
4. Powerfully lift your left knee toward your chest as you squat and stomp your foot down outside the left track.
5. Powerfully lift your right knee high and stomp your foot down inside the tracks.
6. Powerfully lift your left knee high and stomp your foot down inside the tracks.
7. Repeat the sequence 8 to 32 times.

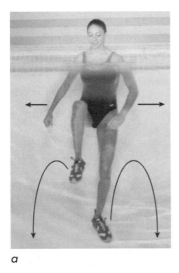
a

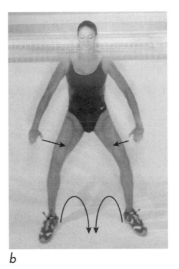
b

Variation: Add arm movements: Push out as you step out and press down as you step in.

Safety Tips: Start with slow movement and build speed as you gain strength and control over the movements. The viscosity of the water makes it difficult to do this movement fast. Maintain your stabilized torso position throughout the move; your stabilization capability determines how fast you can move safely.

CHAPTER 10

Specializing Workouts for Special Needs

The aquatic properties that make water workouts an excellent overall fitness option can greatly benefit people with special health conditions and objectives. Many years of experience have shown that carefully customized water exercise can significantly enhance the health and well-being of pregnant women; older adults; people in rehabilitation for injuries or cardiac recovery; and people with arthritis, fibromyalgia, diabetes, multiple sclerosis, or other movement limitations. Use the guidelines in this chapter to tailor your program to meet your specific needs. Discuss your water workout program with a qualified health, fitness, or wellness professional before you proceed.

Physical Rehabilitation

Water has been used for its healing properties since ancient times. Ancient Roman armies treated wounded soldiers in hot springs. Today, aqua therapy is used to treat people with a wide variety of injuries and conditions. Equipment designers continue to develop innovative ways to take the beneficial properties of water in new directions and to new heights for fitness and rehabilitation.

Water exercise for rehabilitation can be enjoyed by most people, but it is especially well suited for people with joint pain, sport injuries, orthopedic difficulties, weight problems, movement limitations, or lower-back pain. People who derive the greatest benefit include postsurgical patients, chronic pain patients, and elite or avid athletes.

Aqua therapy programs make use of the basic physical properties of water: buoyancy, hydrostatic pressure (which keeps an equal amount of pressure on all of your joints in the water), and viscosity (resistance). Rehabilitative water exercise uses these properties creatively to increase balanced strength and flexibility; to improve coordination, movement skills, and cardiopulmonary functioning (strengthening your heart, lungs, and circulatory system); to retrain your brain and musculoskeletal system in a highly supportive environment; and to promote relaxation and sense of well-being.

Therapists working with recovering individuals use the aquatic environment because the properties of water minimize pressure on all of your joints and muscles. Water makes it possible for people recovering from almost any injury to handle exercise and fitness programs they cannot perform on land, speeding up the often long process of rehabilitation and healing. In addition, the movement of exercise in warm water increases circulation to the injured area, boosting the body's healing mechanisms.

Water offers a safe, protective environment for therapeutic exercise for several other reasons. In water, there is very little negative stress or wear and tear on the body. When you walk on land, there is less resistance to your movement and you are able to swing your arms and move your legs freely. In water, you fight the resistance of the water in order to maintain your balance. By working against the resistance (positive stress) of water, you build strength, coordination, and endurance.

For those who need to lose weight to restore mobility and good health, aquatic rehabilitation makes sense; working out in water burns more calories in less time than performing similar exercise on dry land. A 30-minute workout in water, according to Physical Therapy Forum, can be equivalent to a 45-minute session on land, making water exercise an excellent way to obtain a fat-burning, cardiorespiratory workout on a regular basis.

Key Elements for Water Rehabilitation Exercise

A leading aquatic therapist, Igor Burdenko, recommends a scientific evidence-based approach that emphasizes six essential qualities for effective water therapy: balance, coordination, flexibility, endurance, speed, and strength. Balance enhancement involves use of visualization, challenging your sense of equilibrium and enhancing proprioception, which is your unconscious perception of movement and spatial orientation in response to stimuli within your body. Coordination involves using multiple muscle groups at the same time in movements that simulate normal functional requirements in day-to-day life, such as contracting your abdominals while opening a heavy door or performing the function of a particular sport. Flexibility involves increasing your range of motion by working your joint in multiple directions, such as in the muscle moves in chapter 6, Strengthening and Toning, and the Tai Chi moves in chapter 9, and by cooling and relaxing muscles in lengthened positions, such as in the stretches in chapter 4, Warming Up and Cooling Down, and the yoga positions in chapter 9. Endurance means the number of repetitions that you can perform while still maintaining proper stabilization; build up endurance gradually to prevent reinjury as a consequence of advancing too quickly. Improve your speed by working against the viscosity of water at a gradually increasing tempo over time; the faster you move, the greater is the resistance encountered and the greater the challenge to your stabilizing muscular structures. Gain strength by starting with building a stronger stabilized core at your pelvis, abdominals, back, neck, and shoulders, and then adding peripheral strength in your limbs. To add greater resistance, use your body as a resistance tool against the viscosity of water, and later add resistance and flotation equipment gradually, as described in chapters 6, 7, and 9.

Rehabilitation requires warmer water temperatures (84 to 94 degrees Fahrenheit [29 to 34 degrees Celsius]) and relaxed postures during exercise, which improve circulation to injured areas and promote the healing process. An excellent overall rehabilitation exercise is striding or running forward and backward in an upright position with flotation, without touching the bottom of the pool. Aquatic Tai Chi provides an excellent method for increasing circulation, healing, and range of motion. Rehabilitative water workouts involve natural movements that in some cases can imitate a sport and assist an athlete's recovery of skills that are important for performance. A tennis player, for instance, can practice forehand or backhand racket motion (see Move #45, Sport Training Racket Sweep); a golfer, driving swing; a softball player, the motion of batting, pitching, or catching.

Techniques that build balance use kickboards, water noodles and flotation barbells to support balance and to challenge it as proprioception gains are achieved. To build preliminary postural stability and improve strength around the joints, use flotation and buoyancy equipment to aid in balance and to create resistance during exercises. Improve your balance with Move #55, Bird Dog Point, Move #38, Hip Side Press, and Move #34, Outer- and Inner-Thigh Scissors. Start by holding the pool wall and gradually perform the moves with only fingertips touching the wall, then without touching the pool wall at all. Perform Move #102, Half-Moon Tightrope Touch, first holding onto the pool wall, and then graduate to performing it without touching the wall. Gradually introduce Water Yoga and Water Tai Chi moves from chapter 9, Adding Splash to Workouts. For advanced balance challenges, perform Moves #76, Water Taxi; #75, Kickboard Climb; and #105, Plank and Press. For a focus on rehabilitating, start with the abdominal, back, and lower-body moves in chapter 6, Strengthening and Toning; then build greater core strength in your torso and pelvis by performing Move #54, Plank; #73, Noodle Sidewinder; and #74, Noodle Ring.

Flotation exercise is often used to protect or heal joint and back pain. Flotation exercises create a natural traction on your bones, joints, and connective tissue. The neutral balance position is not possible in a traditional life vest or even in some flotation belts, which create a feeling of being wobbly and unstable, forcing your body to tense. Flotation noodles, the Wet Vest, Wet Vest AT, the HYDRO-FIT Wave belt and the Water Gym belt provide more stable flotation options.

One key guiding factor is avoidance of pain. Forget everything you may have heard about "no pain, no gain." Pain is a signal to stop or change what you are doing. The pain is telling you that the position is wrong, the repetitions too many, the exercise itself too advanced, or the intensity too high; also, you may have overfatigued the affected area with too many workouts. Sometimes the process of finding the right balance requires "detective work": Record your responses to each session, it's content, intensity, and duration. With patience and self-monitoring (listening to your body), you will be able to determine how much is enough; how much is too much, and what kinds of revisions you may need to make to content, form, and technique.

Building up gradually is a second key factor. Instead of working immediately on the injured area, begin by working the muscles around an injury or affected area. Later, when you have gained enough strength so that the surrounding tissues are providing excellent support and the injured area can be worked relatively pain-free, then exercise the injured area.

The third imperative is to work symmetrically, that is, evenly front and back, left and right, top and bottom, and in all other directional nuances. Burdenko explains, "You must work the muscles in all directions to develop harmony. And work simply—simple motion, simple equipment, simple exercise."

The fourth key involves how critical it is to continue to exercise throughout the healing process. In the past, doctors sometimes prescribed complete rest following injury. However, appropriate recuperative exercise produces healing circulation that cannot be generated if you do not combine recovery and rehabilitative exercise with adequate rest.

Common Areas of Injury

The most common types of pain condition, according to insurance and workplace statistics, is back and neck pain. Knee pain comes in third, followed by conditions of the feet, shoulders, hands, and forearms. For specific moves to address particular injuries or pain syndromes, use the tables that follow and Moves #111 to 117 (described in this chapter) for your shoulders, feet, hands, and arms. See table 10.9 for a complete workout to relieve foot pain. Devise a sequence that allows you to heal and strengthen your affected areas, enhances your fitness, and improves your overall well-being. Tables 10.1, 10.2, and 10.3 provide workouts for back and neck, knee, and shoulder pain. The techniques listed are specially selected to provide, for each condition or issue, the appropriate sequences and exercise selections to help you

- warm up without aggravating your condition;
- improve your range of motion and provide stretching that enhances function and decreases pain, starting with the areas distal (farther away) from your affected area;
- strengthen the muscles that are important to the healthy functioning of the area;
- and cool the affected muscles in a lengthened position at the end of the sequence, when they are most receptive to flexibility adaptation.

Table 10.1 The Back and Neck Pain Workout

Thermal Warm-Up (5-10 minutes)	Repeat this Thermal Warm-Up sequence 2-3 times. Move #1 — Water Walk: 1 minute Move #3 — Pomp and Circumstance: 8 times forward, 8 times backward (if balance permits) Move #85 — Arm Circling Move #86 — Scoop the Earth Move #87 — Pat High on the Horse Move #10 — Alternate-Leg Press-Back: 8-16 times, no bouncing. (Perform facing the pool wall or ladder and hold on with both hands. Omit ladder or wall hold if you have neck pain.)
Warm-Up Stretch (5-10 minutes)	Take your time getting into each position and hold each stretch for 10 seconds. It is essential to perform every stretch indicated. Stability is critical, so use the wall for support and follow the instructions for the braced neutral position on pages 19-23 very carefully. If the stretch is uncomfortable, reduce the amount of stretch and double-check your position. Do not use the arm movements designed to keep your body warm. If you get cool, find a warmer pool or wear chlorine-resistant lycra tights or a bodysuit. Stretch #1 — Outer-Thigh Stretch Stretch #2 — Lower-Back Stretch With Ankle Rotation Stretch #3 — Front-of-Thigh Stretch Stretch #4 — Shin Stretch and Shoulder Shrug Stretch #5 — Inner-Thigh Step-Out Stretch #6 — Hip Flexor Stretch Stretch #7 — Straight-Leg Calf Stretch Stretch #8 — Bend-Knee Calf Stretch Stretch #9 — Hamstring Stretch (Repeat previous sequence for other side of body.) Stretch #10 — Deep-Muscle Hip, Thigh, and Buttocks Stretch Stretch #11 — Full Back Stretch (check with your physical therapist) Stretch #12 — Midback Stretch (3 parts) Stretch #13 — Elbow Press-Back Stretch #14 — Shoulder Roll and Chest Stretch Stretch #15 — Chest Stretch Stretch #16 — Upper-Back Stretch Stretch #17 — Torso and Shoulder Stretch Stretch #18 — Shoulder and Upper-Arm Stretch Stretch #19 — Safe Neck Stretch
Aerobic Exercises (1-30 minutes)	Optional. Pick and choose exercises you find comfortable from this list and perform them in the order provided. Move #1 — Water Walk: 1 minute Move #3 — Pomp and Circumstance: 8 times forward, 8 times backward (if balance permits) Move #4 — Knee-Lift Jog or March: March for 15 seconds, no bouncing Move #10 — Alternate-Leg Press-Back: 8-16 times, no bouncing. (Perform facing the pool wall or ladder and hold on with both hands if you don't have neck pain.)

(continued)

Table 10.1 *(continued)*

Aerobic Exercises *(continued)*	Move #12	Snake Walk
	Move #13	Step Wide Side
Flotation Aerobics	Move #26	Aqua Ski
	Move #27	Floating Side Scissors
	Move #28	Back Float Kick and Squiggle
	Move #30	Vertical Flutter Kick
	Move #31	Floating Mountain Climb
	Move #32	Bicycle Pump
	Move #33	Can-Can Soccer Kick
	Move #12	Snake Walk
	Move #13	Step Wide Side
Muscle Strengthening and Toning Exercises	Save abdominal and torso muscle workout moves until last, but before stretching, in order to make sure those muscles are not fatigued during other exercises and can provide the firm contraction your spinal muscles need for adequate protection from injury.	
	Move #34	Outer- and Inner-Thigh Scissors: 8-32 times
	Move #36	Knee Kick: 8-16 times
	Move #37	Runner's Stride: 8-16 times
	Move #38	Hip Side Press: 8-32 times
	Move #39	Pivoted Dip: 4-8 times
	Move #40	Wall Squat: 8-32 times
	Move #42	Calf Lift: 8-16 times
	Move #43	Toe Lift: 8-16 times
	Move #44	Chest and Upper-Back Glide: 8-16 times
	Move #46	Chest and Back Press: 8-32 times
	Move #48	Pivoted Shoulder Press: 8-32 times
	Move #50	Upper-Arm Curl: 8-16 times
	Move #57	Traffic Cop: 8-32 times
	Move #59	Chicken Neck Bob: Gently
	Move #58	Shoulder Shrug and Roll: 8-16 times
	Move #51	Wall-Sit Crunch: Perform 8-16 times with no resistance. Add resistance when you have reached a generally pain-free status.
	Move #54	The Plank: Only when healing has occurred. Should be relatively pain-free.
	Move #104	Diagonal Bicycle Pump: Perform only when you have reached advanced strength.
	Move #106	Otter: Release back and torso tension.
	Move #55	Bird Dog Point: 8-16 times
	Move #56	Cat Back Press: Slowly, 8-16 times
Final Cool-Down Stretches (10 minutes)	Perform the same stretches recommended during Warm-Up, but hold the static stretch positions for 20 to 30 seconds.	

Perform this sequence when you are feeling relatively well. Rest when you are experiencing severe pain. Your doctor may recommend that you use a frozen gel pack on your painful areas before and after exercise to minimize inflammation.

Table 10.2   The Knee Pain Workout

Thermal Warm-Up (5-10 minutes	Perform this Thermal Warm-Up sequence 2 or 3 times.	
	Move #1	Water Walk: 1 minute
	Move #3	Pomp and Circumstance: 8 times forward, 8 times backward
	Move #5	Toy Soldier March: 16 times forward, 16 times backward
	Move #10	Alternate-Leg Press-Back: 8-16 times
Warm-Up Stretch (5-10 minutes)	Take your time getting into each position and hold each stretch for 10 seconds. Perform stretches that can be managed pain free.	
	Stretch #1	Outer-Thigh Stretch
	Stretch #2	Lower-Back Stretch With Ankle Rotation
	Stretch #3	Front-of–Thigh Stretch: Do not bend the knee beyond 90 degrees (right angle).
	Stretch #4	Shin Stretch *Without* Shoulder Shrug
	Stretch #5	Inner-Thigh Step-Out
	Stretch #6	Hip Flexor Stretch
	Stretch #7	Straight-Leg Calf Stretch
	Stretch #8	Bent-Knee Calf Stretch
	Stretch #9	Hamstring Stretch
	(Repeat previous sequence for other side of body.)	
	Stretch #10	Deep-Muscle Hip, Thigh, and Buttocks Stretch
	Stretch #11	Full Back Stretch
	Stretch #12	Midback Stretch (3 parts)
Aerobic Exercises (Optional: 5-30 minutes)	Move #1	Water Walk: 1 minute
	Move #3	Pomp and Circumstance: 8 times forward, 8 times backward
	Move #5	Toy Soldier March: 16-32 times forward and backward
	Move #10	Alternate-Leg Press-Back: 16 times
	Move #13	Step Wide Side: 16-32 times (Keep your knees behind your toes by contracting the front and back of your thighs to stabilize your knee position.)
Flotation Aerobics	Move #26	Aqua Ski: 1-10 minutes (Be sure to keep your legs *straight* but *not locked* during the entire movement.)
	Move #32	Bicycle Pump (Perform slowly and with excellent control.)
	Move #27	Floating Side Scissors: 1-10 minutes
Muscle Strengthening and Toning Exercises	Move #34	Outer- and Inner-Thigh Scissors
	Move #35	Forward-and-Back Leg Glide
	Move #38	Hip Side Press (version 1)
	Add squats, Moves #60-65, gradually as healing progresses	
	Move #42	Calf Lift
	Move #43	Toe Lift
Final Cool-Down Stretches	Perform the same stretches recommended during Warm-Up, but hold the static stretch positions for 20 to 30 seconds.	

Because weight gain is sometimes a factor in knee pain, an optional aerobic section is included. Be sure to include upper-body stretches if you perform upper-body movements. Perform this sequence when you are feeling relatively well. Rest when you are experiencing severe pain. Your doctor may recommend that you use a frozen gel pack on your painful areas before and after exercise to minimize inflammation.

Table 10.3   The Shoulder Pain Workout

Thermal Warm-Up (5-10 minutes)	Repeat this Thermal Warm-Up sequence 2 or 3 times.
	Move #1 — Water Walk: 1 minute
	Move #3 — Pomp and Circumstance: 8 times forward, 8 times backward (if balance permits)
	Move #4 — Knee-Lift Jog or March: March for 15 seconds
	Move #10 — Alternate-Leg Press-Back: 8-16 times
Warm-Up Stretch (5-10 minutes)	Hold each of the stretches for 10 seconds and perform them in the order indicated.
	Stretch #12 — Midback Stretch (3 parts)
	Stretch #13 — Elbow Press-Back
	Stretch #14 — Shoulder Roll and Chest Stretch
	Stretch #15 — Chest Stretch
	Stretch #16 — Upper-Back Stretch
	Stretch #17 — Torso and Shoulder Stretch
	Stretch #18 — Shoulder and Upper-Arm Stretch
	Stretch #19 — Safe Neck Stretch
Exercises for Range of Motion and Muscle Strengthening	Perform these exercises slowly. Start with a low number of repetitions and build gradually.
	Move #44 — Chest and Upper-Back Glide: 4-32 times
	Move #46 — Chest and Back Press: 4-32 times
	Move #47 — Diagonal Front Shoulder- Press: 4-32 times
	Move #48 — Pivoted Shoulder-Press: 4-32 times
	Move #49 — Side Arm Pump: 4-32 times, both variations
	Move #50 — Upper-Arm Curl: 4-32 times
	Move #57 — Traffic Cop: 4-32 times
	Move #58 — Shoulder Shrug and Roll: 4-32 times
Final Cool-Down Stretches (10-15 minutes)	Perform the same stretches recommended during Warm-Up, but hold the static stretch position for 20 to 30 seconds.

The sequence illustrated is designed to help alleviate shoulder pain. Start with no equipment. As the routine begins to feel easy, gradually add webbed gloves, then paddles, and then non-flotation bells. To obtain a well-rounded workout, you may wish to include additional exercises from "The Back and Neck Pain Workout."

Pregnancy

Keeping in shape during pregnancy can have several benefits. During pregnancy, a woman can anticipate a gradual potential weight gain (ideally) of 20 to 25 pounds, with its inevitable stress on the back. Pregnant women need muscle strengthening exercise to help them carry their increased body weight better and, after the birth, to help them carry the baby. Some physicians formerly discouraged weight training for fear of injuries because of softening of the ligaments and changes in the body's center of gravity that are associated with pregnancy. However, current studies of muscle strengthening during pregnancy show that such injuries are rare, probably because women who experience joint pain or balance problems stop whatever is causing them discomfort.

Labor itself presents a physical challenge of substantial proportions for most women. With a first pregnancy, women can expect to spend an average of 17 hours in labor. Women who have been exercising during pregnancy enjoy greater endurance and stamina during labor, are less likely to require medical intervention, and enjoy a quicker return to prepregnancy fitness levels following the birth. After the birth, mothers who exercised during pregnancy may be able to handle the stresses of motherhood better than women who avoided physical activity.

Studies by Dr. Robert G. McMurray examined the effects of land-based and water exercise on pregnant women. Exercising in the water reduced thermal stress, keeping the future mother's temperature within safer levels for the fetus, and reduced her blood pressure and heart rate. The buoyancy of the water unloads the weight of the pregnancy, making exercise a much more comfortable choice for pregnant women.

Water also eliminates the danger of jumping or jarring. The cushioning, cooling effects of water make aquatic aerobic activity ideal for pregnant women. Although water minimizes the potentially hazardous effects of overexertion during pregnancy, it is still very important to warm up and cool down gradually. Breathing fully and evenly encourages proper oxygen delivery to your system.

Pregnant women who wish to engage in prenatal exercise activities should have the approval of their medical caregivers. Unless a woman has a history of miscarriage or spontaneous abortion, is experiencing vaginal bleeding, or has some other serious medical condition, exercise should become a routine from the beginning of pregnancy or, better yet, prior to pregnancy. According to Barbara B. Holstein, MS, of the International Childbirth Education Association, exercise delivers real bonuses for pregnant women: It reduces many of the common discomforts of pregnancy, helps prepare the mother-to-be for the rigors of birth, and eases the postpartum experience. Holstein has identified several specific benefits:

1. Exercise improves circulation and builds muscular strength, which in turn reduces the pain, discomfort, and severity of varicose veins, commonly suffered by pregnant women.

2. Exercise can help correct posture problems associated with pregnancy and prevent back pain by reducing muscular imbalance and enhancing strength.

3. Exercise can alleviate the discomfort and immobility of swollen joints by increasing circulation, thereby abating the edema (swelling caused by collection of fluids in the tissues) brought on by pregnancy.

4. Exercise can ease digestive discomforts and constipation.

5. Exercise with a flexed ankle instead of pointed toes can reduce leg cramps. Flex at the ankle by lifting your toes toward your shin.

6. Exercise strengthens the abdominal and thigh muscles, which are essential during the second stage of labor (when the baby passes through the birth canal).

7. Firm abdominals return to normal more readily after childbirth. Additionally, exercise helps women cope with postpartum "baby blues."

8. Exercise helps a pregnant woman feel good about herself and move with grace and greater ability.

List adapted from B.B. Holstein, 1998, "Shaping up for a healthy pregnancy" (Champaign, IL: Human Kinetics), 5:36-40; 47-55.

Certain activities can be beneficial during pregnancy, while others should be avoided. The American College of Obstetricians and Gynecologists has developed a number of guidelines for pregnant women to follow when exercising.

ACOG Guidelines

The American College of Obstetrics and Gynecology describes water exercise activity as "great for your body because it works so many muscles. The water supports your weight so you avoid injury and muscle strain. It also helps you stay cool and helps prevent your legs from swelling." ACOG recommends the following guidelines for women who are pregnant.

Exercise Routine

- Exercise during pregnancy is most practical during the first 24 weeks. During the last 3 months, it can be difficult to do many exercises that once seemed easy. This is normal.

- If it has been some time since you've exercised, it is a good idea to start slowly. Begin with as little as 5 minutes of exercise a day and add 5 minutes each week until you can stay active for 30 minutes a day.

- Always begin each exercise session with a warm-up period for 5-10 minutes. This is light activity, such as slow walking, that prepares your muscles. During the warm-up, stretch your muscles to avoid stiffness and soreness. Hold each stretch for at least 10-20 seconds.

- After exercising, cool down by slowly reducing your activity. This allows your heart rate to return to normal levels. Cooling down for 5-10 minutes and stretching again also helps you to avoid sore muscles.

Things to Watch

The changes your body is going through can make certain positions and activities risky for you and your baby. While exercising, try to avoid activities that call for jumping, jarring motions or quick changes in direction that may strain your joints and cause injury.

Warning Signs

Stop exercising and call your doctor if you get any of these symptoms:

- Vaginal bleeding
- Dizziness or feeling faint
- Increased shortness of breath
- Chest pain
- Headache

- Muscle weakness
- Calf pain or swelling
- Uterine contractions
- Decreased fetal movement
- Fluid leaking from the vagina

There are some risks from becoming overheated during pregnancy. This may cause loss of fluids and lead to dehydration and problems during pregnancy. When you exercise, follow these general guidelines for a safe and healthy exercise program:

- After the first trimester of pregnancy, avoid doing any exercises on your back.
- Avoid brisk exercise in hot, humid weather or when you have a fever.
- Wear comfortable clothing that will help you to remain cool.
- Wear a bra that fits well and gives lots of support to help protect your breasts.
- Drink plenty of water to help keep you from overheating and dehydrating.
- Make sure you consume the daily extra calories you need during pregnancy.

While you exercise, pay attention to your body. Do not exercise to the point that you are exhausted. Be aware of the warning signs that you may be overdoing it. If you notice any of these symptoms, stop exercising and call your doctor.

American College of Obstetricians and Gynecologists. Exercise during pregnancy. ACOG Patient Education Pamphlet AP119. Washington, DC: ACOG; 2003.

Exercise and Sport Physiology During Pregnancy

Most experts recommend exercise prior to pregnancy; if you start out in good shape, you'll have an easier time staying in shape. Sport Gynecologist Mona Shangold suggests that, for women with normal, uncomplicated pregnancies, it is "probably reasonable to continue exercising at the same level of exertion you are accustomed to before pregnancy, but it may not be safe to exercise more vigorously or more frequently than that."

The same level of exertion may not mean the same level of intensity or frequency. You may have to make adjustments to your exercise program as the pregnancy progresses to compensate for weight gain. The additional weight increases your workload, so you may need to reduce the intensity and the frequency of exercise in order to continue exercising at the same level of exertion you did before you gained the weight. Good news for pregnant women is that, according to the research of Dr. James Clapp, a woman's cardiopulmonary capability is greatly enhanced during pregnancy and remains so postpartum; a mother who has recently given birth can deliver more oxygen to the working muscles per heartbeat than she did before pregnancy. The dilemma is to find a realistic way to maintain that fitness advantage along with all of the other challenges of being mother to a newborn.

Ratings of perceived exertion—that is, judging by how you feel—may be a safer means of measuring your aerobic intensity level than monitoring your heart rate. The International Association of Fitness Professionals recommends use of the perceived exertion scale (page 11) because it encourages you to take note of how hard your changing system is working. Or use the Talk Test to keep your activity within aerobic intensity limits: If you cannot carry on a slightly breathy conversation during exercise, you are exercising too hard.

Your pregnant body still sends you signals, although it may not say the same things it did during your prepregnancy workouts. High-spirited physical enthusiasm usually gives way to the wisdom that it is best not to push it. If you are planning on becoming pregnant, practice listening to your body's signals; if you have learned to listen to your nonpregnant body, your pregnant body will provide you with important information as well.

Pregnancy Workout

Moderation is the key for any prenatal exercise program. Maternal pulse and blood pressure rise more quickly during exercise, and, while you are adapting to all of the changes that your body is going through, you may not be able to deliver oxygen to your working muscles as quickly as usual. You may fatigue more quickly as a result. Sudden bursts of high-energy exercise or prolonged workouts are inappropriate. Follow the adage, "If it hurts, don't do it."

Eat a small, nutritious snack (low fat, high fiber, complex carbohydrate; avoid refined flours and sugars) about an hour before you exercise and a well-balanced meal after you are through. Limiting food intake so that you burn your body's own stores is absolutely not appropriate; it can be detrimental to the fetus.

Holstein recommends the following guidelines:

- Avoid rapid twisting movements, jumps, or rapid shifts in direction, level, or speed.
- Exclude any exercises that cause hyperextension of any joint or flexion taken beyond the maximum point of resistance.

- Avoid letting your back sag or arch.
- Eliminate exercises that require you to bend forward at the hip with a straight back. If both feet are on the floor, forward flexion should always be performed with bent knees.

List adapted from B.B. Holstein, 1998, "Shaping up for a healthy pregnancy" (Champaign, IL: Human Kinetics), 5:36-40; 47-55.

Use the Pregnancy Workout version of the Basic Water Workout routine in table 10.4 and concentrate on making adjustments based on the previous recommendations. Stop any exercise that feels uncomfortable or painful.

Your exercise sequences should emphasize movements that strengthen your back and abdominal muscles. The Lunge and moves such as the Alternate-Leg Press-Back are particularly helpful because they strengthen your muscles while promoting balance and alignment. Eliminate fast turning motions in side and forward lunges. Use the wall for balance and stability as appropriate on any given day—some days will feel more or less challenging than others.

Use the Final Cool-Down section to teach your mind and body to relax, as well as to maintain flexibility. Tension reduction skills and the ability to relax consciously come in handy during childbirth when you need to relax during labor contractions. You can develop basic relaxation skills by focusing your attention on softening the muscles involved in each stretch. Consciously allow the muscle fibers to unwind, and breathe deeply. Imagine that you can bring your breath right to the muscle you are relaxing; exhale deeply. This method of "conscious release" can be used for every part of your body and helps you eliminate tightness and tension. Use pleasant, soothing instrumental music. You may wish to perform these relaxation exercises outside the pool in a lounge chair under warm towels if your body feels too cool.

Creative Moves for Exercise During Pregnancy

To add more interest or challenge to the basic pregnancy workout, see the moves in chapter 7, Intensifying Workouts, and chapter 9, Adding Splash to Workouts. Choose moves that adhere to Holstein's guidelines presented earlier in this section. If you have been performing similar moves prior to pregnancy, you can mix these moves into your sequence for variety or higher intensity:

- Power Squat Moves, #60 through 65
- #74 Noodle Ring (similar to Pilates moves)
- Water Tai Chi, Moves #82 through 88
- Water Yoga, Moves #94 through 100
- Water Yoga Booty Ballet, Moves #107 through 110

If you are having trouble with your ankles and feet, follow the water workout guidelines for plantar fasciitis in table 10.9.

Table 10.4   Pregnancy Workout

Thermal Warm-Up (5 minutes)	Start slowly and build very gradually.	
	Move #2	Pedal Jog: 30 seconds
	Move #3	Pomp and Circumstance: 8 times in each direction
	Move #1	Water Walk: Stride slowly for 60 seconds
	Move #4	Knee-Lift Jog or March: 15 seconds as a nonbouncing march
	Move #10	Alternate-Leg Press-Back: 16 times
	Move #12	Snake Walk: Slowly for 2 minutes
Warm-Up Stretch (5 minutes)	Stretch #1	Outer-Thigh Stretch
	Stretch #2	Lower-Back Stretch with Ankle Rotation
	Stretch #3	Front-of-the-Thigh Stretch
	Stretch #4	Shin Stretch and Shoulder Shrug
	Stretch #5	Inner-Thigh Step-Out
	Stretch #6	Hip Flexor Stretch
	Stretch #7	Straight-Leg Calf Stretch
	Stretch #8	Bent-Knee Calf Stretch
	Stretch #9	Hamstring Stretch
	(Repeat previous sequence for other side of body.)	
	Stretch #10	Deep-Muscle Hip, Thigh, and Buttocks Stretch
	Stretch #11	Full Back Stretch
	Stretch #12	Midback Stretch (eliminate the first position)
	Stretch #13	Elbow Press-Back
	Stretch #14	Shoulder Roll and Chest Stretch
	Stretch #15	Chest Stretch
	Stretch #16	Upper-Back Stretch
	Stretch #17	Torso and Shoulder Stretch
	Stretch #18	Shoulder and Upper-Arm Stretch
	Stretch #19	Safe Neck Stretch
Aerobic Exercises	Warm up gradually, maintain a moderate pace, and cool down slowly.	
	Move #2	Pedal Jog: 30 seconds
	Move #3	Pomp and Circumstance: 8 times in each direction
	Move #1	Water Walk: 60 seconds
	Move #4	Knee-Lift Jog or March: 15 seconds as a nonbouncing march
	Move #10	Alternate-Leg Press-Back: 16 times
	Move #13	Step Wide Side: 8 times in each direction
	Move #12	Snake Walk: 1-2 minutes
	Flotation Exercises: Use two empty plastic water jugs, water noodle, or upper-arm flotation cuffs.	
	Move #26	Aqua Ski: 10-30 seconds
	Move #27	Floating Side Scissors: 10-30 seconds
	Move #29	Vertical Frog Bob: 8 times
	Move #30	Vertical Flutter Kick: 10-30 seconds

Aerobic Exercises *(continued)*	Move #31	Floating Mountain Climb: 30-60 seconds
	Move #32	Bicycle Pump: 10-30 seconds
	Move #33	Can-Can Soccer Kick: 10-30 seconds
	Move #12	Snake Walk: 1-2 minutes
	Move #13	Step Wide Side: 8 times right, 8 times left. Repeat.
	Move #10	Alternate-Leg Press-Back: 16 times
	Move #4	Knee-Lift Jog or March: 15-30 seconds as a nonbouncing march
	Move #1	Water Walk: 1-2 minutes
	Move # 3	Pomp and Circumstance: 8 times each direction
	Move #2	Pedal Jog: 30 seconds
Muscle Strengthening and Toning Exercises (5-10 minutes)	Begin with fewer repetitions and add more as the weeks progress.	
	Move #51	Wall-Sit Crunch: 8-16 times
	Move #53	Sitting V: 6-16 times
	Move #34	Outer- and Inner-Thigh Scissors: 8-16 times
	Move #35	Forward-and-Back Leg Glide: 8-16 times per side
	Move #36	Knee Kick: 8-16 times per side
	Move #38	Hip Side Press: 8 times
	Move #40	Wall Squat: 8-16 times
	Move #42	Calf Lift: 8-16 times
	Move #43	Toe Lift: 8-16 times per foot
	Move #44	Chest and Upper-Back Glide: 8-16 times
	Move #46	Chest and Back Press: 8-16 times
	Move #48	Pivoted Shoulder Press: 8-16 times
	Move #49	Side Arm Pump: 4-8 times
	Move #50	Upper-Arm Curl: 8-16 times
	Move #58	Shoulder Shrug and Roll: 4-8 times each
	Move #55	Bird Dog Point: 8-16 times
	Move #56	Cat Back Press: 8-16 times
Final Cool-Down Stretches (10-15 minutes)	Repeat Warm-Up Stretch sequence, but hold each stretch for 20-30 seconds. Add this Final Cool-Down Stretch:	
	Stretch #19	Safe Neck Stretch

Older Adults

Adults in the prime of life need more time to warm up and must cool down more gradually. As we get older, sudden strenuous exercise can be hazardous to the heart. Thermal Warm-Up of 10 to 15 minutes at the beginning of your aerobic sequence, which extends the aerobic warm-up by 5 to 10 minutes, helps prepare your joints and muscles for greater exertion and gradually increases your circulation and heart rate. Add more striding forward and back, as well as sideways, and more repetitions of the remainder of the warm-up moves in your sequence, and move at a pace that allows you to maintain your musculoskeletal stability and to breathe fully and deeply. This adjustment prevents fatigue, soreness, and injury after exercise. Strength training is also important for older adults, so include 8-10 strengthening and toning exercises with 10-15 repetitions of each exercise two or three times per week. And, to decrease risk of falling, perform balance exercises in your routine as well.

During the Water Aerobics section, warm up slowly, and then continue to build very gradually and monitor your intensity, working toward a moderate level of perceived exertion. Decrease intensity when it is warranted by taking smaller steps, reducing resistance (for example, sliding through the water with a slicing hand position instead of cupped hands), moving more slowly, and minimizing bouncing and bounding. Use these same techniques to cool down at the end of your Water Aerobics segment. Abrupt cessation of vigorous exercise can cause pooling of blood in your limbs, which places unnecessary strain on your heart while your body works to divert the blood back to your trunk. To prevent this unwanted stress on your cardiovascular system, gradually reduce intensity during the cool-down period at the end of Water Aerobics over at least 10 minutes. By cooling down gradually, you can also prevent muscle soreness after exercise.

Regulating body temperature can be more challenging for older adults. If you tend to chill easily, wear a chlorine-resistant, long-sleeved top and tights or a neoprene jacket (see page 31). Drink plenty of cool (but not cold) water before, during, and after your workout to help regulate your body temperature effectively and to prevent early onset of fatigue. Icy water can be more difficult to absorb and can cause cramping.

A fully rounded workout helps you improve or maintain flexibility; keeps you strong and physically independent; improves the health and longevity of your heart, lungs, and circulatory system; and gives you renewed energy and vigor. Proper exercises for body posture, warm-up, cool-down, and flexibility, as described in the Basic Water Workout, help prevent muscle soreness.

To increase variety and depth in the Basic Water Workout, add the following moves:

- Water Country Line Dancing, Moves #77 through 81
- Water Tai Chi, Moves #82 through 88
- Water Yoga, Moves #94 through 100

For those at a more advanced level of fitness, build on the Basic Water Workout by concentrating on moves that challenge your core strength and build muscle strength and tone:

- Strengthening and Toning Moves, chapter 6
- Power Squat Moves, #60 through 65
- #72 Water Bug Belly Crunch, #73 Noodle Sidewinder, and #74 Noodle Ring

If you are just getting back into shape, you may choose to start your new water workout program with a sequence that does not include aerobic conditioning until you strengthen your muscles a bit. (See "Initial Conditioning Stage," pages 18 and 19.) A beginning sequence of this type may include Thermal Warm-Up, Warm-Up Stretch, Strengthening and Toning Moves, and Final Cool-Down Stretches. After you gain a sense of balance and strength in the water, add an Aerobic Moves section of about 5 to 10 minutes. Follow the Water Workout for Older Adults format described in table 10.5, and plug in your favorite exercises from the Basic Water Workout descriptions. Use the nonbouncing, low-impact variation of each exercise. If one exercise doesn't feel right, try another until you find one you like. Perform all of the stretching exercises and stretch only to the comfortable point of resistance.

Table 10.5   Water Workout for Older Adults

Thermal Warm-Up (10 minutes)	Choose the workout intensity that is right for you at your current level of fitness. Older adults come in all shapes, sizes and fitness levels, and many of us are more active and mobile than ever. Water walking is an excellent warm-up for almost everyone, including older adults. Concentrate on using proper body alignment. Walk slowly forward and backward and Pedal Jog lightly. Omit backward walking if it feels like you might fall over. Use aqua shoes or an old pair of lightweight canvas sneakers to improve traction, stability, and movement confidence. Water Tai Chi moves provide an excellent thermal warm up, enhance range of motion, quiet the mind, and improve body awareness.
Warm-Up Stretch (5 minutes)	Complete the entire stretch sequence. Study and emulate the position instructions carefully and avoid stretching beyond a comfortable and normal range of motion. You may wish to eliminate the "keep warm" upper- and lower-body motions in order to focus on your stretch stability. Therefore, try to locate a pool environment that you find comfortably warm. Water Yoga moves are a good option for increasing flexibility, range of motion, and relaxation.
Water Aerobics (Build up to 20-30 minutes)*	Start out slowly and use the first 10 minutes to elevate your intensity gradually to a moderate, comfortable level. Monitor your intensity carefully. If you are just beginning an exercise program, or have back or neck pain, avoid impact in your movements by eliminating hops, bounces, and jumps. During the last 10 minutes, gradually lower your intensity until your breathing is smooth, even, and unlabored. Eliminate any aerobic exercises that feel too strenuous or uncomfortable. Build to a longer duration over a period of months if weight control is an objective.
Strengthening and Toning Exercises (10-15 minutes)	Perform each of the exercises in a steady, controlled manner. Start with 8 repetitions of each exercise and build to 16 or more over a period of months or years. Pay close attention to your body position and stability. Eliminate any exercises that feel uncomfortable and try them again at a later date when you are stronger and have developed greater range of motion.
Final Cool-Down Stretches (10-15 minutes)	Complete all of the Final Cool-Down Stretches, checking your position to ensure proper body alignment. Hold each stretch for 10 to 30 seconds. If a stretch position is uncomfortable, check your position again and ease up on the stretch by reducing the extent or degree of the stretch. For instance, if your calf feels tight during a Calf Stretch, bring your front and back feet a bit closer to reduce the stretch. If it still causes discomfort, eliminate that particular stretch and try it at a later date when your flexibility improves overall.

*You have the option of starting out with 5-10 minutes of aerobic exercise and gradually adding a minute each week.

You need a day of rest between bouts of exercise to build your strength and prevent pain or injury from overuse. Exercise every other day, starting with 5 to 10 minutes if you have been inactive for a number of years, and add a minute each week until you reach a period of time you find comfortable. A good objective for cardiovascular health and overall fitness is to start out with 10 minutes per bout and build toward 30 minutes of aerobic exercise per session. Adding even a few minutes at a time can effectively improve your cardiovascular health. Begin each session with Thermal Warm-Up and Warm-Up Stretches; finish every workout with a thorough stretch routine that includes all of the stretches in chapter 4, Warming Up and Cooling Down. If you have been exercising regularly, nearly every day, go ahead and dive into a daily water exercise routine, but give your body a chance to adapt gradually to the new challenges presented by the physical properties of water. You will be surprised how easy the exercise feels while you are in the water and how heavy a workout you realize you have had later on, after you have been out of the water for a while.

Cardiac Recovery

People at risk of cardiac disturbance require longer warm-up and more gradual cool-down periods. Cardiac rehabilitation professionals strongly recommend that you train aerobically 3 to 5 days each week. If may be necessary to lower the intensity and duration of your aerobic training, in which case you need to exercise 4 to 6 times per week and eventually increase the duration of your workouts.

To promote injury-free functioning, your workout should include strength training and flexibility work as well as aerobic or cardiovascular exercise. Focus on breathing fully throughout your workout. Use "belly breathing," in which you expand your whole belly when you breathe rather than just your ribs and chest. To help develop your ability to belly breathe, practice pushing your belly against your waistband when you inhale. Strive to breathe in an even rhythm. (Research suggests that the most efficient breathing rate during vigorous aerobic exercise is about 30 breaths per minute.) Although no exercises in this book include exertions that require holding your breath (the Valsalva maneuver), you should avoid any tendency to hold your breath, especially when holding a squeezed or contracted muscle, and stay away from activities such as isometrics, holding up heavy objects, or pressing against a wall. Those maneuvers elevate blood pressure and can trigger a cardiac event. While contracting a muscle to work on muscle strength, use "straw breathing:" Inhale deeply and blow out through pursed lips as you squeeze the muscle firmly.

Experts agree that a well-rounded cardiac recovery program (including cardiorespiratory conditioning, strength training, and flexibility exercise) as soon as possible after surgery can help prepare patients to return to work and leisure activities. The basic components of a training session for people with cardiac recovery appear in table 10.6. Noted cardiac rehabilitation researchers

Table 10.6 Basic Components of a Cardiac Training Session

Component	Duration
Thermal Warm-Up	10 minutes
Warm-Up Stretch	10 minutes
Muscular Conditioning	10 minutes
Aerobic Exercise (mild intensity with very gradual warm-up and very gradual cool-down)	5-60 minutes
Cool-Down (stretch for flexibility)	5-10 minutes

Pollock, Wilmore, and Fox suggest that the first 6 to 8 weeks of your recovery exercise program should be monitored by cardiac medical professionals.

Qualified health professionals can determine whether you have health factors that require exercise restrictions. They can devise the right exercise program for your health situation and keep track of your exercise responses to ensure that you are on the right program.

Cardiac Recovery Workout

Cardiologists and researchers at the University of Rhode Island Human Performance Laboratory have revealed valuable information regarding the thermal qualities, adjustable intensity, and improved dynamics of water for cardio-respiratory fitness. Their carefully monitored scientific studies of water-versus land-based exercise revealed previously undocumented factors that may make water exercise a superior avenue for cardiac rehabilitation exercise.

Water-based exercise was shown to produce lower incidence of arrhythmias, or irregular heartbeat, which can signal cardiac disturbances. The mitigating factor is water temperature. As a result of their findings, University of Rhode Island researchers recommend exercising in water at what they call "thermoneutral temperature." During vertical aerobic exercise, thermoneutral water temperature is usually 83 to 86 degrees Fahrenheit (28 to 30 degrees Celsius).

Cardiac arrest and other major cardiovascular events are not common in cardiac rehabilitation programs. The best way to handle potential emergency situations is to exercise under qualified supervision. To prevent medical emergencies, your health professional can help you monitor your heart rate, blood pressure, and work intensity and guide you through the progressive phases of recovery. Once you have progressed beyond the three medically established initial phases of recovery, you can continue your water workout program on your own and check in periodically for evaluation. Return for professional exercise evaluation whenever you change your exercise routine.

Before you begin your workout, check the pool temperature to ensure that it is between 83 and 86 degrees Fahrenheit (28 to 30 degrees Celsius). Follow the Cardiac Recovery Workout sequence in table 10.7. Start with very moderate intensity levels and short duration. During the Aerobic Exercise, warm up

Table 10.7   Cardiac Recovery Workout

Thermal Warm-up (10-15 minutes)	Move slowly and build very gradually.	
	Move #2	Pedal Jog: 30 seconds
	Move #3	Pomp and Circumstance: 8 times in each direction
	Move #1	Water Walk: Stride slowly for 60 seconds
	Move #4	Knee-Lift Jog or March: 30 seconds as a nonbouncing march
	Move #9	Heel Jacks: 8 times
	Move #10	Alternate-Leg Press Back: 8 times
	Move #12	Snake Walk: Very slowly for 2 minutes
Warm-Up Stretch (5-10 minutes)	Hold each stretch position for 10 seconds and breathe deeply.	
	Stretch #1	Outer-Thigh Stretch
	Stretch #2	Lower-Back Stretch With Ankle Rotation
	Stretch #3	Front-of-the-Thigh Stretch
	Stretch #4	Shin Stretch and Shoulder Shrug
	Stretch #5	Inner-Thigh Step-Out
	Stretch #6	Hip Flexor Stretch
	Stretch #7	Straight-Leg Calf Stretch
	Stretch #8	Bent-Knee Calf Stretch
	Stretch #9	Hamstring Stretch
	(Repeat previous sequence for other side of body.)	
	Stretch #10	Deep-Muscle Hip, Thigh, and Buttocks Stretch
	Stretch #11	Full Back Stretch
	Stretch #12	Midback Stretch
	Stretch #13	Elbow Press-Back
	Stretch #14	Shoulder Roll and Chest Stretch
	Stretch #15	Chest Stretch
	Stretch #16	Upper-Back Stretch
	Stretch #17	Torso and Shoulder Stretch
	Stretch #18	Shoulder and Upper-Arm Stretch
	Stretch #19	Safe Neck Stretch
Muscle Strengthening and Toning Exercises	Begin with fewer repetitions and add more as the weeks progress. Breathe deeply during every exercise.	
	Move #50	Wall-Sit Crunch: 8-16 times
	Move #52	Floating Curl: 8-16 times
	Move #34	Outer- and Inner-Thigh Scissors: 8-16 times
	Move #35	Forward-and-Back Leg Glide: 8-16 times per side
	Move #36	Knee Kick: 8-16 times per side
	Move #39	Pivoted Dip: 4-8 times per side
	Move #42	Calf Lift: 8-16 times
	Move #43	Toe Lift: 8-16 times per foot
	Move #44	Chest and Upper-Back Glide: 8-16 times
	Move #46	Chest and Back Press: 8-16 times
	Move #47	Pivoted Shoulder Press: 8-16 times
	Move #49	Side Arm Pump: 4-8 times
	Move #50	Upper-Arm Curl: 8-16 times
	Move #58	Shoulder Shrug and Roll: 4-8 times each
	Move #55	Bird Dog Point: 8 times

Aerobic Exercises	Start with 5 minutes and gradually build to 30 minutes over a period of 15 weeks. Your physician may recommend gradually lengthening the aerobic duration to an hour or more. With each workout, begin the aerobic section slowly, build progressively to a moderate aerobic exertion, and then gradually decrease intensity.
	Move #2 Pedal Jog: 30 seconds
	Move #3 Pomp and Circumstance: 8 times in each direction
	Move #1 Water Walk: 60 seconds
	Move #4 Knee-Lift Jog or March: March for 30 seconds
	Move #9 Heel Jacks: 8 times
	Move #10 Alternate-Leg Press-Back: 8 times
	Move #12 Snake Walk: 1-2 minutes
	Move #13 Step Wide Side: 8 times in each direction
	Move #14 Hydro Jacks: 8-16 times
	Move #15 Cross-Country Ski: 16 times
	Move #16 Sailor's Jig: 8-16 times
	Move #25 Jump Twist: 8 times
	Move #26 Aqua Ski: 10-30 seconds
	Move #27 Floating Side Scissors: 10-30 seconds
	Move #28 Back Float Kick and Squiggle: 10-30 seconds
	Move #30 Vertical Flutter Kick: 10-30 seconds
	Move #31 Floating Mountain Climb: 30-60 seconds
	Move #32 Bicycle Pump: 10-30 seconds
	Move #33 Can-Can Soccer Kick: 10-30 seconds
	Move #12 Snake Walk: 1-2 minutes
	Move #13 Step Wide Side: 8 times right, 8 times left. Repeat.
	Move #10 Alternate-Leg Press-Back: 8 times
	Move #9 Heel Jacks: 8 times
	Move #4 Knee-Lift Jog or March: March for 15-30 seconds
	Move #1 Water Walk: 1-2 minutes
	Move #3 Pomp and Circumstance: 8 times in each direction
	Move # 2 Pedal Jog: 30 seconds
Final Cool-Down Stretches (10 minutes)	Repeat Warm-Up Stretch sequence, but hold each stretch for 20 to 30 seconds.

Warm up very gradually, maintain a moderate pace, and cool down very slowly.

very slowly, building intensity very gradually. Then use a long aerobic cool-down, while gradually reducing your exertion, slowly decreasing intensity, and returning to a resting heart rate.

To build on your cardiac recovery workout, add challenge in *one fitness dimension at a time:* once you have mastered your current level, increase, at a rate of about 5 percent, either frequency, intensity, or duration. Duration is the best place to begin, but change it over time in order to give your body differing challenges, and use very small increments of increase. This gradual increase gives your body a chance to adapt to the increased challenge while reducing the risk of negative cardiac events. Cut back on your intensity, duration, or frequency if you are feeling tired. Most often, if you are feeling unwell, it is wisest to wait until you feel better to begin exercising again. When you return to your water workouts, start at a somewhat lower level than you were accustomed to prior to your hiatus and then gradually increase the level over time.

Arthritis

More than 670 million people worldwide, or 10 percent of the world's population, have arthritis according to Glenn McWaters, author of *Deep Water Exercise for Health and Fitness.* Because hydrodynamics reduces joint stress and weight bearing, exercise performed in the water is considered one of the most universally beneficial methods of managing all types of arthritis.

There are more than 100 different kinds of arthritis. Most are characterized by inflammation of the joints, which causes painful swelling and can result in loss of joint motion or function. With proper diagnosis and treatment, joint damage caused by arthritis can be limited or prevented, and joint motion and flexibility can be improved. Because of the fact that there are many ways to minimize pain and loss of motion from arthritis, people with arthritis need to work with qualified health and fitness professionals to determine the treatment program that is best for them. Most experience relief with regular water activity. In fact, water activity is considered the best therapy for osteoarthritis or rheumatoid arthritis, according to Edward A. Abraham, orthopedic surgeon and author of *Freedom from Back Pain.*

Pain in your joints may make you want to hold them very still. But not using your joints causes the joints, ligaments, and muscles to lose range of motion and to weaken over time. Immobility may also cause your muscles to shorten and tighten up, causing you to feel more pain and stiffness and limiting your ability to do the things you want to do.

Regular exercise helps keep the joints moving. It restores and preserves flexibility and strength and can protect against further damage. Because exercise helps improve coordination, endurance, and mobility, it makes you feel good about yourself and your ability to accomplish more. Water provides a comfortable way for people with arthritis to exercise gently and without pain. The buoyancy of the water supports the body, lessens stress on the joints, and frees movement for greater range of motion. Water also acts as a force of resistance to help build muscle strength.

If you have arthritis, strive to exercise daily for approximately 45 minutes to maintain and improve flexibility, strength, and endurance; 15 minutes 3 times a day may work better in many cases than 45 minutes all at once. To achieve maximum benefit, fully submerge the joints you are working. Submerging the joint relieves it from the stress of gravity, and the buoyancy should help you move that part of your body through its full, normal range of motion. Exercise intensity should be determined by the level of pain tolerance you may be experiencing on any given day. Actively inflamed joints may become worse with excessive exercise; therefore, reduce exercise greatly during inflammatory episodes.

Here are some special precautions recommended by the Arthritis Foundation:

- Consult your doctor to determine whether water exercises are appropriate for you.

- Be sure that someone else is nearby to help you in and out of the pool, if necessary.

- Check the temperature before entering the pool. The water temperature should feel soothing and comfortable, not hot. Temperatures between 83 and 88 degrees Fahrenheit (28 to 31 degrees Celsius) are appropriate for exercisers with arthritis.

- If you feel light-headed or nauseated, carefully get out of the water immediately.

- If joint swelling, stiffness, or pain increases, discontinue exercise and consult your doctor.

- Never enter a pool after using alcohol or drugs. The sleepiness, drowsiness, and raised or lowered blood pressure that can result could cause injury or even death. If you are taking medication, consult your doctor before entering the pool to exercise.

- Start slowly and don't overdo it. Learn to recognize your body's reactions to exercise and stop activities before you become fatigued. Arthritis symptoms flare up and disappear over time, so exercises that feel easy one day may feel difficult the next. Change your exercise program so that it takes your current symptoms into account.

- Pay close attention to pain signals. If you continue to exercise when you feel pain, you may cause further damage.

If warm water makes your arthritis feel better, this is the best workout for you. Make sure the pool temperature is 83 to 88 degrees Fahrenheit (28 to 31 degrees Celsius) before you enter the water. Relax and enjoy the soothing sensation of the water. When your muscles and joints feel comfortable and free of tension, begin your exercise routine slowly. Give yourself enough time after exercising to relax your muscles completely before you get out of the water. You can exercise in warmer water if no aerobic exercise is planned.

The Arthritis Foundation provides important guidelines for water exercise:

- Submerge the body part that you plan to exercise.
- Move that body part slowly and gently.
- Breathe in a normal, deep rhythmic pattern and avoid holding your breath.
- Start and finish with simple exercises.
- Alternate between difficult and simple activities to minimize fatigue.
- Use flotation devices to help conserve your energy.
- Do not add resistance equipment unless a health professional has instructed you to do so. If you use resistance equipment at all, employ low-resistance versions.
- Avoid gripping the pool edge or equipment tightly. Hold on to the pool wall gently or place your elbow on the edge to improve stability during wall exercises.
- Move through the complete range of motion around your joint. Do not force movement. Stop if you feel sudden or increased pain.
- Complete 3 to 8 repetitions, based on what works best for you. Over time, gradually increase the number of repetitions to 15 if you tolerate the increase well.
- If a particular exercise is uncomfortable for you, don't do it. If it hurts, stop.
- Pain that lasts for more than 1 or 2 hours after exercise may signal overuse. Cut back the next time you exercise. If pain persists after cutting back, change the exercise.
- Begin gradually and slowly. Don't overdo. Do not perform more repetitions than you are comfortable with.
- If you have severe joint damage or joint replacement, check with your doctor or surgeon before you do any of the exercises.

The exercise program in table 10.8 can be performed while you are standing or sitting in the pool or using flotation equipment. For detailed instructions on the exercises, see chapters 4, 5, and 6. Include Move #111, Shoulder Circles, if you have pain in your shoulder, upper back, or neck and Moves #112 to 117 if arthritis affects your hands, arms, or feet.

Table 10.8 Arthritis Workout

Thermal Warm-Up (5 minutes)	Choose one or more of the following:	
	Move #1	Water Walk
	Move #4	Knee-Lift Jog or March
	Move #5	Toy Soldier March
	Move #13	Step Wide Side
Warm-Up Stretch (5 minutes)	Complete all of the stretches that you find comfortable. Hold each stretch lightly for 10 seconds. Stretching should *never* be painful.	
	Stretch #1	Outer-Thigh Stretch
	Stretch #2	Lower-Back Stretch with Ankle Rotation
	Stretch #3	Front-of-the-Thigh Stretch
	Stretch #4	Shin Stretch and Shoulder Shrug
	Stretch #5	Inner-Thigh Step-Out
	Stretch #6	Hip Flexor Stretch
	Stretch #7	Straight-Leg Calf Stretch
	Stretch #8	Bent-Knee Calf Stretch
	Stretch #9	Hamstring Stretch
	(Repeat previous sequence for other side of body.)	
	Stretch #10	Deep-Muscle Hip, Thigh, and Buttocks Stretch
	Stretch #12	Midback Stretch (3 parts)
	Stretch #13	Elbow Press Back
	Stretch #14	Shoulder Roll and Chest Stretch
	Stretch #15	Chest Stretch
	Stretch #16	Upper-Back Stretch
	Stretch #17	Torso and Shoulder Stretch
	Stretch #18	Shoulder and Upper-Arm Stretch
	Stretch #19	Safe Neck Stretch
Aerobic Exercises with Flotation (5-15 minutes)	This segment is optional and should be performed only when you are not tired. Remember, warm up and cool down gradually and perform the exercises at the speed that feels most comfortable to you. Use a flotation belt, vest, upper-arm cuffs, or water noodle.	
	Move #26	Aqua Ski
	Move #27	Floating Side Scissors
	Move #29	Vertical Frog Bob
	Move #32	Bicycle Pump

(continued)

Table 10.8   *(continued)*

Exercises for Range of Motion and Strengthening (15-20 minutes)	Move #34	Outer- and Inner-Thigh Scissors
	Move #35	Forward-and-Back Leg Glide
	Move #36	Knee Kick
	Move #37	Runner's Stride
	Move #38	Hip Side Press
	Move #39	Pivoted Dip
	Move #40	Wall Squat
	Move #44	Chest and Upper-Back Glide
	Move #46	Chest and Back Press
	Move #47	Diagonal Front Shoulder Press
	Move #48	Pivoted Shoulder-Press
	Move #49	Side Arm Pump
	Move #50	Upper-Arm Curl
	Move #57	Traffic Cop
	Move #58	Shoulder Shrug and Roll
	Move #111	Shoulder Circles
	Move #42	Calf Lift
	Move #43	Toe Lift
	Move #112	Toe Curl
	Move #113	Ankle Alphabet
	Move #114	Ankle Inversion and Eversion
	Move #115	Finger Curl
	Move #116	Finger Touch
	Move #117	Thumb Circle
	Move #56	Cat Back Press
Final Cool-Down Stretches (10 minutes)	Perform the same stretches recommended during Warm-Up, but hold the static stretch positions for 20 seconds.	

MOVE 111   SHOULDER CIRCLES

Purpose: This move is intended to relax the tension around your shoulder joint, which can aggravate pain in your shoulder, neck, or upper back. It improves your range of motion around the shoulder capsule and prevents pain.

Starting Position: Stand with your left side next to the pool wall, in water just below shoulder depth. Place your left foot forward and your right foot back. Place your left elbow and forearm on the pool edge, or place your left hand on your left thigh, and let your right arm hang down toward the floor.

Action:

1. Circle your arm slowly, from the shoulder, in small, counterclockwise circles and then in clockwise circles.

2. Turn around and repeat using the other arm. Repeat 4 to 32 times in each direction with each arm.

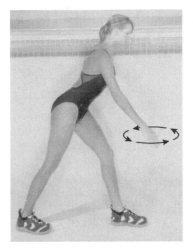

Variation: Shoulder retraction helps strengthen the stabilizer muscles that keep your shoulder blade back and down, thereby protecting your joint from poor biomechanics—that is, using your shoulder in a bad position. Start in the same position, but allow your arm to drop down toward the pool bottom from your shoulder; then use the muscles around your shoulder blade to draw your shoulder back into a neutral, stabilized position. Keep your arm straight, and use your shoulder blade muscles exclusively. Use a small motion that isolates the muscles that draw your shoulder back. Avoid hunching your shoulder up toward your ear.

Safety Tips: Move very slowly within your pain-free range of motion. Increase the diameter of the circle over time as your range of pain-free motion increases. Reduce the diameter if and when you have a flare-up and the pain-free zone decreases.

TOE CURL

MOVE
112

Purpose: This move relieves foot pain, relaxes tension in your foot, strengthens the muscles that work your toes and the sole of your foot, and improves the range of motion in your foot.

Starting Position: Stand next to the pool wall, in waist- to chest-deep water, and hold on to the edge to support your balance. Stand upright in the neutral position with your abdominal and buttocks muscles firmly contracted. You may need to take off your aqua shoes for this exercise.

Action: Raise one knee so that your foot is off the ground. Curl your toes down and then straighten them out. Imagine you are picking up a towel with your bare foot.

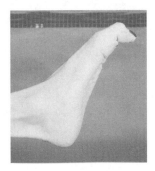

Variation: You can also perform this move sitting on pool steps or in the bathtub or hot tub.

Safety Tips: Move slowly, smoothly, and deliberately. Exercise one foot at a time.

ANKLE ALPHABET

Purpose: This move relieves pain in your foot, ankle, or lower leg; helps you regain or preserve range of motion in your ankle; strengthens your ankles and feet; and reduces "foot drop" that causes your toes to stick to the floor, leading to tripping.

Starting Position: Stand next to the pool wall, in waist- to chest-deep water, and hold on to the edge to support your balance. You may need to take off your aqua shoes for this exercise.

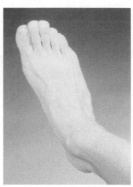

Action: Raise one knee so that your foot is off the ground. "Write" the alphabet with your toes, moving your ankle through all of its ranges of motion. Exercise one foot at a time.

Variation: You can also perform this move sitting on pool steps or in the bathtub or hot tub.

Safety Tip: Move slowly, smoothly, and deliberately.

ANKLE INVERSION AND EVERSION

Purpose: This move relieves pain in your foot, ankle, or lower leg; helps you regain or preserve range of motion in your ankles; strengthen your ankles and feet; and prevents ankle "turns" that weaken the integrity of your ankle joint.

Starting Position: Stand next to the pool wall, in waist- to chest-deep water, and hold on to the edge to support your balance. You may need to take off your aqua shoes for this exercise.

Action:

1. Raise one knee so that your foot is off the ground.

2. Think of your ankle as a door hinge and your foot as the door, and slowly rotate your foot inward at the ankle so that your instep is higher than the outside of your foot (figure *a*).

3. Slowly rotate your foot outward so that your instep is lower than the outside of your foot (figure *b*).

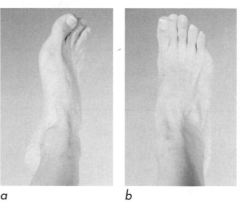

a   *b*

Variation: You can also perform this move sitting on pool steps or in the bathtub or hot tub.

Safety Tips: Move slowly, smoothly, and deliberately. Exercise one foot at a time.

FINGER CURL

Purpose: This move helps you overcome hand pain, improves your pain-free range of motion, and enhances manual dexterity.

Starting position: Place your hand in a body of water. Use warm water if you have arthritis symptoms.

Action: Open and close your palms slowly. Make a loose fist (figures *a*, *b*).

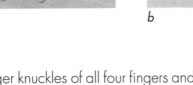

a   b

Variations:

- Bend the larger knuckles of all four fingers and bring your fingertips toward the tops of your palms.
- Close and open your hand one finger at a time.

Safety Tip: Move slowly and increase the range of motion gradually.

FINGER TOUCH

Purpose: This move helps you overcome hand pain, improves your pain-free range of motion, and enhances manual dexterity.

Starting position: Place your hand in a body of water. Use warm water if you have arthritis symptoms.

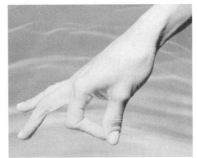

Action: Touch the tip of your thumb to each of your fingers one at a time.

Safety Tip: Move slowly and increase the range of motion gradually.

MOVE 117 THUMB CIRCLE

Purpose: This move helps you overcome hand pain, particularly in your thumb joint; improves your pain-free range of motion, and enhances manual dexterity.

Starting position: Place your hand in a body of water. Use warm water if you have arthritis symptoms.

Action: Make slow, large circles with your thumb, in both directions.

Safety Tip: Move slowly and increase the range of motion gradually.

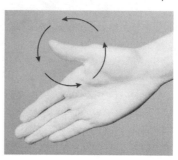

To tailor your sequence, or to add interest and challenge to the basic Arthritis Workout, include some of the following moves:

- Water Tai Chi, Moves #82 through 88
- Water Yoga, Moves #94 through 100
- Power Squat Moves, #60 through 65, performed very slowly
- #72 Water Bug Belly Crunch, #73 Noodle Sidewinder, and #74 Noodle Ring, performed very slowly
- #106 Otter

Fibromyalgia

Although it may seem like a very difficult thing to do when you suffer from this fatigue-producing condition, the right kind of exercise has proven to be one of the best treatments for people with fibromyalgia. Fibromyalgia is a chronic condition, sometimes considered a form of arthritis, characterized by multiple symptoms, including widespread pain, intense fatigue, stiffness, and muscle weakness. People with this condition have higher amounts of the neurotransmitters that signal pain responses and lower amounts of natural pain killers, such as serotonin. This means that sufferers experience chronic aches and pains, interrupted sleep, and other symptoms that can make life feel nearly impossible.

With the pain and fatigue of fibromyalgia, exercise and many daily activities get reduced or stopped completely. Inactive muscles atrophy and are more prone to trauma and dysfunction. The many necessary hormones that should be released during exercise and daily physical activities do not respond reliably and consistently in fibromyalgia sufferers.

People with fibromyalgia have had difficulty finding effective treatment solutions, contributing to the severe frustration caused by the illness. However, research evidence shows that exercise can actually help decrease pain symptoms and improve the quality of life for people with fibromyalgia. It is often assumed that fibromyalgia and exercise don't go together because of the chronic pain associated with fibromyalgia syndrome. In truth, an appropriate fibromyalgia exercise program, consistently followed, relieves pain, strengthens connective tissue, and increases flexibility and blood flow.

Water is one of the best environments for a fibromyalgia exercise program. Water exercise improves muscle flexibility and strength in an environment that reduces discomfort caused by fibromyalgia. If you have fibromyalgia, it is crucial to get your muscles healthy; that in itself can offer some relief. Muscles that are flexible allow a healthy range of motion around the joint. The importance of muscle strength is apparent to everyone with fibromyalgia every day, when daily tasks become more of a challenge, especially during flare-ups. The stronger you are, the more you can move around each day.

Aerobic exercise in particular has been shown to curtail fibromyalgia symptoms. Water exercise may be best tolerated because it supports the body and cushions muscles and joints. Walking back and forth in the water provides a challenging workout that does not overstress your body. For some, completely eliminating impact shock is necessary, and, in that case, flotation aerobic moves are the best choice. Water temperature is important. Avoid extremely warm or cold water, which may make symptoms worse.

Although it may be difficult to start and maintain an exercise program, depending on the severity of your pain, if you stay with it and modify it according to your level of symptoms, you will begin to notice many benefits. With fibromyalgia, exercise plays a key role in healing because a properly designed exercise routine can help in many ways because it:

- decreases muscle weakness and improves strength;
- strengthens connective tissue (ligaments and tendons) while enhancing muscle tone;
- makes muscles feel less stiff, especially in the morning and after physical exertion;
- increases flexibility, allowing for a fuller range of motion without pain, strain, pulls, and tears;
- often improves sleep patterns (in the case of aerobic exercise), making it easier to fall asleep and stay asleep, which, in turn, reduces overall fibromyalgia symptoms;
- helps reduce pain, because it causes the release of endorphins, the body's natural painkillers;
- increases blood flow to working tissue, which transports oxygen and healing nutrients to the muscles;
- increases endorphins released by the hypothalamus, healing and uplifting with natural pain-relieving and sleep-deepening effects and

alleviating some of the anxiety, depression, and pain associated with fibromyalgia;

- stimulates the production of serotonin and growth hormone, the exact pain-reducing and muscle-repair hormone imbalances linked with individuals who have fibromyalgia;
- enhances production of T-cells from the thymus, making a greater number of cells that boost the immune system available to the body;
- relieves negative stress, increases energy, and reduces fatigue;
- promotes weight loss, thus reducing strain on the joints; and
- increases bone mass and reduces risk of fracture or osteoporosis.

Fibromyalgia Workout

If you haven't been active, consult your health care professional before you start any type of exercise program in order to avoid injury or exacerbation of symptoms. It is extremely important to introduce aerobic exercise into your routine slowly. Start out slowly and gently and very gradually build up your duration, intensity, frequency, and amount of resistance. Always begin with a warm-up. Do several minutes of slow walking, followed by 3 to 5 minutes of careful stretching, to get your muscles warmed up and ready for exercise. Always finish with a thorough stretch routine.

If you are just starting out begin with 5 minutes of aerobic activity and then slowly add 1 minute at a time, building up the length of your workout until you can complete 30 minutes, 2 or 3 times a week. You can perform the warm-up and stretch sequence every day and achieve significant benefits.

Expect to feel some pain and stiffness when you first begin to work out, but remember that these symptoms fade as your body becomes accustomed to activity. Learn to distinguish the difference between muscle soreness and aggravation of fibromyalgia pain. If pain after exercise is deep and lingering, fibromyalgia symptoms have likely been aggravated, and you may need to trim back your intensity, duration, or frequency. Muscle soreness, on the other hand, is not debilitating, and simply refers to the feeling that your muscles have worked harder than usual, so there may be a small amount of discomfort for a few hours or up to a day or so. Always set aside some time to rest and recuperate after you exercise.

The hardest part of exercising with fibromyalgia is the frustration of knowing that you used to be able to do more. Channel that frustration into your workouts and remind yourself that, every time you move around, you are improving. Taking control of your health can bring tremendous relief, both physically and emotionally.

Perform the Arthritis Workout, focusing especially on stretching, breathing, and relaxing, as well as walking and cycling motions, all of which relax tense muscles, improve circulation, deliver nutrients to the working muscles, and enhance range of motion. Flotation aerobics, such as deep-water running with a flotation belt, are a good choice because they completely eliminate impact shock. Water Tai Chi, found on page 171 in chapter 9, offers an ideal range-of-motion and strength-building workout style for people with fibromyalgia.

Plantar Fasciitis

Plantar fasciitis causes stabbing or burning pain in the heel or sole of the foot and is usually worse in the morning when you first step out of bed. The fascia tighten overnight and can become aggravated after activities such as walking, running, tennis, or dancing, especially on hard surfaces. People with very flat feet or very high arches are more prone to plantar fasciitis. This injury affecting the sole or flexor surface (plantar) of the foot happens when overuse causes inflammation of the tough, fibrous band of tissue (fascia) connecting the heel bone to the base of the toes (see figure 10.1). It often feels like a stone bruise when it first begins.

In most cases, you can avoid surgery or other invasive treatments to overcome the pain of plantar fasciitis by taking steps to prevent plantar fasciitis from recurring. Rest, ice, elevation, and careful stretching, often over weeks or months, depending on how long you have had the condition, can counteract the affects of overuse and eliminate pain. Use a frozen gel ice pack on your heel and the soles of your feet several times a day for 10 to 20 minutes at a time to reduce inflammation and relieve pain.

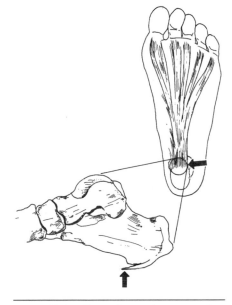

Figure 10.1 Plantar fasciitis happens when overuse causes inflammation of the tough, fibrous band of tissue (fascia) connecting the heel bone to the base of the toes.

Reprinted, by permission, from L. Micheli, 1996, "Healthy runner's handbook" (Champaign, IL: Human Kinetics), 104.

Water workouts are an excellent form of exercise for overcoming plantar fasciitis because of the reduced or eliminated impact shock and the advantageous environment for non-weight-bearing stretching, particularly in the lower leg and foot. Other activities need to be curtailed while you are overcoming plantar fasciitis. Self-care is important and should be initiated as early in the onset of symptoms as possible because you can develop other problems with your foot, knee, hip, and back because of the way that plantar fasciitis changes how you walk. Avoiding impact shock and engaging in daily stretching can prevent this exacerbation. In addition to your lower leg and foot, stretching the muscles of your hips, thighs—particularly the hamstrings—back, sides, and abdomen are also key elements for managing plantar fasciitis in order to prevent the spread of pain to other parts of the body. Table 10.9 provides a workout designed for plantar faciitis.

Table 10.9 Plantar Faciitis Workout

Thermal Warm-Up (5 minutes)	Move #1	Water Walk
	Move #3	Pomp and Circumstance
Warm-Up Stretch (5 minutes)	Hold each stretch position for 10 seconds. Perform each stretch that is included in the "Basic Starter Workout," with special attention to the following stretches:	
	Stretch #2	Lower-Back Stretch with Ankle Rotation
	Stretch #4	Shin Stretch and Shoulder Shrug
	Stretch #7	Straight-Leg Calf Stretch
	Stretch #8	Bent-Knee Calf Stretch
	Stretch #5	Inner-Thigh Stretch
	Stretch #1	Outer-Thigh Stretch
	Stretch #3	Front-of-the-Thigh Stretch
	Stretch #9	Hamstring Stretch
Aerobic Moves (Start with 5 minutes and gradually increase to 30 minutes or more)	Avoid jumping moves until you are not experiencing a flare-up, are fully healed, and your plantar fasciitis symptoms are no longer aggravated by jumping.	
	Move #1	Water Walk, in multiple directions, front, side, and backward.
	Move #10	Alternate-Leg Press-Back
	Move #13	Step Wide Side
	Move #12	Snake Walk
	Perform any of the flotation aerobic moves.	
Water Tai Chi and Water Yoga	As you become less symptomatic, use any and all of the Water Yoga and Tai Chi moves to improve and maintain strength and flexibility of the muscles of your feet and legs and to protect your back and knee health.	
Muscles Strengthening and Toning Exercises	Include any and all Strengthening and Toning Moves, when you are relatively symptom free, but concentrate on the following:	
	Move #112	Toe Curl
	Move #42	Calf Lift
	Move #43	Toe Lift
	Move #113	Ankle Alphabet
	Move #114	Ankle Inversion and Eversion
	Move #40	Wall Squat
	Move #41	Squat Touch
	Move #39	Pivoted Dip
	Move #55	Bird Dog Point
Final Cool-Down Stretches (10 minutes)	Repeat the entire Warm-Up Stretch sequence, but hold each stretch longer, for 20 seconds.	

The order of exercises here is designed to allow for stretching of the muscles next to the main area affected before stretching those directly associated with flexibility in the plantar fascia, located on the heel and sole of the foot. In addition, stretches that represent greater challenge for the muscles that control the sole of the foot are placed last in the sequence, in order to be sure that those muscles are stretched and ready for their stabilization role.

Multiple Sclerosis

Therapeutic water exercise is recommended for people with multiple sclerosis because it improves control over the functional motion of your body. Water workouts can help people with multiple sclerosis to maintain or improve physical mobility, increase range of motion and flexibility, gain muscle strength, improve balance and coordination, and manage stress. Water exercise can help ease the symptoms of multiple sclerosis when certain precautions are taken. The most important thing is not to overdo it. If you stretch too far or too long or work your muscles too hard, you can end up straining an already compromised muscular system, increasing your pain and causing your body and mind to become overstressed, overworked, and overtired.

Pushing too hard can bring on symptoms and hasten progression of the disorder. Be patient with yourself; some days are much better than others. Staying physically active helps you have a greater percentage of good days, and water exercise is the ideal soothing and supportive environment for enhancing fitness when you have multiple sclerosis.

Check with your doctor or physical therapist before you begin in order to gain recommendations about what exercises, intensity, and duration are right for your current symptoms and goals.

Safety Tips

- Always warm up gradually at the beginning and cool down at the end of your workout.
- If you plan to work out for 30 minutes, start with 10-minute workout sessions and very gradually work your way up over several weeks or more.
- Avoid slippery floors, poor lighting, throw rugs, and other potential hazards that cause slipping and tripping.
- If you have difficulty balancing, exercise within reach of the edge of the pool, a grab bar, or rail.
- If, at any time, you feel sick or you begin to feel pain, stop.
- If you are sensitive to heat—your symptoms either reappear or become worse when your body heat rises—do the following:
  - Avoid exercise during the hot time of the day (10 a.m. to 2 p.m.). Exercise in the morning or evening if you are exercising outside.
  - Drink plenty of fluids, especially water.
  - Become aware of your body. If you notice any symptoms that you didn't have before you began exercising, slow down or stop exercising until you cool down.

After an easy, fluid-movement range-of-motion warm-up and light stretching, begin a striding workout. Begin at level one by standing as upright as possible and begin stride walking with assistance. The gliding action of striding in water—with the assistance of holding on to the pool edge, guide bar, or, better yet, a trusted person holding onto your hands in front of you and walking backward (you determine the pace)—can soothe tense muscles, enhance balance, and improve range of motion for walking.

When you have become proficient at assisted stride walking and are having a good day, go on to level two: Use your best stabilized upright posture and walk with a long-handled flotation bell or a water noodle (or two noodles together) held in front of you. For greater stability and balance assistance, use the Water Walking Assistant equipment referred to in chapter 2 on page 35.

On your very good days, once you are proficient at level two, try level three: striding with two flotation bells or water noodles, one in each hand, held at your sides. If the balance required is too much, return to level two or one.

Healthy postural alignment is an important goal for people with multiple sclerosis; it can be addressed with water striding and by performing the Back and Neck Pain Workout provided earlier in this chapter. If you have experienced injuries, include the injury-specific moves in chapter 10 that apply to your situation. Review the exercise recommendations with your doctor or physical therapist to make sure that they are right for you. Then follow the exercise sequence appropriate for your needs 2 or 3 times per week, taking at least one day of rest between workouts to ensure healing. Gradually build your duration and intensity as your condition improves, and reduce intensity, duration, and even frequency when you experience flare-ups. The format of the Arthritis Workout on pages 227-228 is appropriate for people with multiple sclerosis; it provides excellent exercises for enhancement of your range of motion, gentle moves of aerobic endurance that also assist with core strength, and joint-friendly techniques for strengthening your muscles. Water Tai Chi and Water Yoga represent some of the best workout moves for overcoming spasticity, building muscular strength, and enhancing range of motion. Add these moves to your multiple sclerosis water workout once you feel comfortable in the water and are ready to add a new dimension to your workout.

To order a National Multiple Sclerosis Society video titled *Aqua Exercise for Multiple Sclerosis*, contact distributor Sprint Rothhammer. The 18-minute video demonstrates an active water workout with exercises to reduce spasticity, build muscles, and improve posture and body alignment.

Diabetes

Regular physical activity is very important for people with diabetes because it helps control blood glucose levels, increase energy levels, improve heart health, and promote emotional well-being. As long as there are no other medical complications to contraindicate exercise, most people with type 1 and type 2 diabetes can benefit from at least 30 to 60 minutes of physical activity on most days of the week. Always consult your healthcare team before beginning a new exercise program.

Type 1 Diabetes

For people with type 1 diabetes, exercise has many positive health benefits, including short-term blood glucose control. Because exercise typically has the effect of lowering blood glucose, people with type 1 diabetes need to monitor carefully their blood glucose levels before, during, and after exercise. Also important is keeping an appropriate snack or beverage nearby to prevent blood sugar emergencies.

Although exercise generally has the effect of lowering blood glucose, it is important to note that, for some people with type 1 diabetes, an intense workout can actually cause high blood sugar, particularly if blood glucose levels were high prior to the workout. For safe exercise with type 1 diabetes, an essential element of your fitness plan is to monitor glucose levels before and after working out and to log your glycemic response to various physical activities. Use these results to adjust your program to fit your specific needs.

Type 2 Diabetes

Inactive lifestyle is a major risk factor for developing type 2 diabetes, and the high incidence of obesity and overweight among people with type 2 is also highly associated with lack of physical activity. According to the American Diabetes Association, starting a regular workout program can reduce body mass and consequently decrease the insulin resistance of type 2 diabetes. Research studies have shown that people with type 2 diabetes who exercise regularly have better hemoglobin A1c profiles than those who do not exercise, indicating that diabetes comes under better control with regular exercise. Along with nutrition and healthy eating improvements, exercise is priority one in controlling type 2 diabetes. In some cases, these lifestyle changes can eliminate the need for medication altogether.

Exercise is also a key tool in preventing one of the leading complications of type 2 diabetes—heart disease. American Diabetes Association guidelines indicate that regular activity lowers triglyceride levels and blood pressure, two of the most important factors for preventing heart disease.

Diabetes Workout

The goal of a workout for people with either type 1 or type 2 diabetes is to keep body weight down and blood sugar steady. If you are introducing water exercise after a period of inactivity, begin with water walking three times a week. Include a thermal warm-up of light activity, followed by a warm-up stretching routine of about 5 to 10 minutes, and finish with a thorough cool-down stretch sequence of another 5 to 10 minutes. Regardless of how hard you plan to exercise, be sure to warm up and stretch. As you begin to find water walking easier, start expanding on your water workout routine. Follow the guidelines for the Arthritis Workout or the Basic Starter Workout. Start slowly and build very gradually over time. It may work best to begin with 5 minutes and add 1 minute each day. Flotation aerobic exercise offers a great way to reduce risk of irritation and injury to your feet.

Always use aqua shoes to protect your feet and make sure that they fit well; people with diabetes are much more vulnerable to foot and skin injuries, and even a small skin irritation that you may not feel because of your diabetes can become a major problem, in some cases leading to amputation. Always wear an identification tag indicating that you have diabetes, to ensure proper treatment if there is a problem when you are exercising.

For Experienced Exercisers with Diabetes

Are you diabetic and athletic? Push the training envelope by performing advanced power moves (chapter 7, Intensifying Workouts). Challenge yourself with high-intensity, deep-water running and other flotation aerobic moves (chapter 5, Benefiting From Aerobic Moves). Strengthen your core with Noodle Moves from chapter 9, Adding Splash to Workouts. People with diabetes who are athletic must watch especially carefully for foot and skin injuries that can be caused by intense exercise. In particular, plyometric jumping moves can be damaging to the skin of the feet. Although the water provides a safer environment than land for athletes who seek to enhance performance with plyometrics, people with diabetes must use extreme caution and extremely high-quality, well-fitting protective footwear if they are going to engage in water plyometrics.

Managing Diabetes With Exercise

Sometimes it may seem easier to take a pill, or even a shot, than to exercise. But the truth is that exercise, in combination with healthy eating, is one of the best things you can do to take care of yourself if you have diabetes. Water exercise offers a great solution for people with diabetes because it protects your feet (always wear aqua shoes), takes the weight off your joints, and makes exercise fun rather than a chore. The benefits of regular, appropriate exercise for people with diabetes are many:

- It burns calories and improves body composition, which quickens your metabolism and helps you lose weight or maintain a healthy weight.
- It helps your body respond to insulin and can be effective in managing your blood glucose levels.
- It can lower your blood glucose and possibly reduce the amount of medication you need to treat diabetes.
- Combined with healthy eating, exercise can control type 2 diabetes in some people without the need for medications.
- Exercise improves your circulation, especially in your arms and legs, where people with diabetes can have problems with serious consequences.
- It reduces stress, which can raise your glucose level.

Strive to exercise at the same time every day for the same duration. This regularity helps control your blood sugar levels. Exercise at least three times a week for about 30 to 60 minutes, and develop a plan that will help you build to 5 or 6 times per week. If you plan to exercise more than 1 hour after eating, eat a high-carbohydrate snack, such as 6 ounces of fruit juice or a rice cake without topping. If you have not eaten for more than 1 hour or if your blood sugar is less than 100 to 120, eat or drink something like an apple or a cup of soy milk before you exercise. Carry a snack with you in case of low blood sugar.

If you use insulin, exercise after eating, rather than before. Test your blood sugar before, during, and after exercising. Do not exercise when your blood sugar is higher than 240. If you are not an insulin user, test your blood sugar before and after exercising if you take pills for diabetes. If your blood sugar level is over 300 mg/dl, do not exercise. Also, if you are at your peak medication level, it is better not to exercise. Whether or not you take insulin, do not exercise if you are sick, short of breath, have ketones in your urine, or are experiencing any tingling, pain, or numbness in your legs.

If you feel your blood sugar lowering, eat something right away. Don't wait. According to the American Diabetes Association, it is important to treat the symptom when you feel it. Exercise makes your body more sensitive to insulin, so it is crucial to monitor your blood sugar carefully before and after your workout. Eat a snack beforehand, and pack some fuel to go: Take some raisins, a banana, or pretzels with you to raise your blood glucose level if necessary.

The bottom line is, you can gain better control over your diabetes, instead of your diabetes controlling you, when you make water exercise a regular habit, monitor your blood sugar, change and adapt your eating and medication as needed (with the help of your doctor), and manage stress effectively.

Your Personal Fitness Profile

Date: _____

1. **What is your body type?** Think about what your body was like as a child or adolescent.

   ❏ **Ectomorphic.** Long and lanky, small-boned, with limbs longer in relation to the trunk. Muscles are not naturally well defined.

   ❏ **Endomorphic.** Body is rounded and curvy or pear-shaped, with soft, rounded shoulders and wider hips. Limbs are shorter relative to the trunk.

   ❏ **Mesomorphic.** Muscular physique, or builds muscle easily. May be broader at the shoulders and hips, narrower at the waist. When weight is gained due to excess intake or lack of activity, body fat tends to gather at the waist or abdomen.

   ❏ **Endo-mesomorphic.** Naturally strong muscles with a tendency to carry more weight in the hips and thighs.

   ❏ **Ecto-mesomorphic.** Thin and wiry with well-defined muscles. If weight is gained due to excess intake or lack of activity, body fat tends to be gained around the middle.

   ❏ **Endo-ectomorphic.** Tend to put on body fat in the hips and thighs, while also being long-limbed and small-boned. Upper body may be slender and trunk longer than average.

For each body type or combination, follow the fitness tips described in chapter 8 under Alterations for Specific Body Types on page 153.

2. **Measure your aerobic endurance.** Warm up for 5 minutes with water walking and stretch each muscle group. Next, mark the time and see how long you can continue to water walk without losing proper water walking form (see Move #1 Water Walk). Be sure to start the aerobic sequence with a low intensity warm up, build to peak aerobics (water run, if you are ready), and finish with lower intensity. This measured duration will be your baseline: Start with an aerobics sequence that lasts this number of minutes. Once you feel masterful completing that number of minutes, and it feels pretty easy to complete the full baseline time, it will be time to increase your time by 10 percent.

   My Baseline Number of Aerobic Minutes:_____

3. **Examine your degree of flexibility.** Stand upright facing the pool steps, or stand facing the pool wall. Lift one leg and place it on the highest step or highest point on the wall where you can keep your leg straight, your back flat, and remain standing upright. Be sure to keep your abdominal muscles contracted firmly to protect the lower back.

_____ My leg and torso make a 90 degree angle. (You have healthy flexibility—stretching will help maintain it).

_____ My leg and torso make a wider than 90 degree angle. (Flexibility will be a very important focus in customizing your water workout).

_____ My leg and torso make a smaller than 90 degree angle. (You are very flexible. Stretch lightly to maintain flexibility, and consider focusing on strengthening to improve joint stability).

4. **Measure your balance.** Stand with your side to the pool wall in waist to chest deep water and time how long you can stand on one foot in the stork position without touching the pool wall. Remove aqua shoes (if appropriate for you) and place your hands on your hips, then place one foot against the inside knee of your supporting leg. Be sure to stand upright with your chest lifted, shoulder blades back and down, and your abdominal muscles contracted—Balance and stabilization go hand-in-hand. Raise the heel to balance on the ball of the foot. Time yourself from the time of heel raise until one of the follow occurs:

- hands come off the hips.
- supporting foot swivels or moves or hops in any direction.
- non-supporting foot loses contact with the knee.
- heel of the supporting foot touches the floor.

How many seconds did you complete?

❏ **Fair = less than 24.** Enhance your balance practicing Move #34 Outer/Inner Thigh Scissors without touching the pool wall, or with only fingertips touching the pool wall. Perform Move #98 Half Moon, first holding onto pool wall, then graduate to performing it without touching the wall. Gradually introduce Water Yoga and Water Tai Chi moves from chapter 9.

❏ **Average = 25 to 39.** Maintain your balance skills by performing water walking with arms out to your sides, or hands on hips. Increase the challenge by water walking with eyes closed. Water Yoga will advance your balance skills.

❏ **Good = 40 to 50.** Maintain or increase your balance skills with Pilates Move #101 The Saw. Challenge yourself with Water Yoga.

❏ **Excellent = more than 50.** Challenge your balance with Move #105 Plank and Press and with Plyometric Moves in chapter 7, Intensifying Your Workouts.

5. **Identify your coordination skill.** Stand about an arm's length from the pool wall. Contract your abdominal muscles and keep your shoulder blades back and down. Push your right leg back and bring your left arm forward, similar to Move #15, Cross-Country Ski, but with no jumping. Time yourself to see how many seconds you can properly bring your right leg back at the same time you bring your left arm forward, and your left

leg back at the same time you bring your right arm forward. Stop the clock the first time that your body gets confused about which leg goes back and which arm goes forward.

How many seconds did you complete?

❏ **Fair or Beginner = Fewer than 20.** Enhance your coordination by performing Moves #55, Bird Dog Point, Move #34, Outer- and Inner-Thigh Scissors, Move #35, Forward-and-Back Leg Glide, and Move #38, Hip Side Press. Hold on to the pool wall with one arm, and move your other arm through the water in opposition to the direction of your leg movement. Perform Flotation Aerobics Move #26, Aqua Ski, and focus on moving your right leg back while your left arm moves forward, and your left leg back, while your right arm moves forward.

❏ **Average = 20 to 30.** Maintain and build your coordination abilities by performing aerobics moves in waist- to chest-deep water. Use alternate arm and leg motions.

❏ **Good = 40 to 50.** Maintain and build coordination by performing Move #20, Mogul Hop, and Plyometric Move #67, Hurdle Hop, while focusing on using your arms in opposition to your legs. Challenge your fine motor coordination by performing the Country Line Dancing Moves #77 to 81.

❏ **Excellent = More than 50.** Maintain and enhance your coordination skills by performing Move #62, Squat Knee Lift, Move #63, Squat Knee Curl, and Move #64, Squat Scissor Lift. Strengthen large movement coordination with Moves #69, Plyometric Jack, #70, Plyometric Ski, and the explosive coordination moves of Water Kickboxing, Moves #89 to 93. Sharpen your fine motor skills with Country Line Dancing Moves #77 to 81.

6. **Track your speed.** Warm up and stretch. Using excellent postural form in your water walking, time how long it takes you to walk the length of your pool. If you have only deep water, time yourself for how long it takes you to walk or run the length of the pool using a flotation belt or vest. Record the time here and measure yourself a month from now, after you have been engaging in water workouts regularly. Self-tracking encourages you to give yourself a pat on the back for your progress. If your speed has not improved, focus on improving your core strength, employ interval training during your aerobic sequence (walk for 2 minutes and then run or walk quickly for 2 minutes), or, if you are quite fit, add resistance equipment to your feet and hands during the aerobics sequence in shallow water or in deep water with flotation.

_____ Minutes to cross the length of the pool

Your Fitness Personality

How do you create a fitness plan that is right for you? Begin by asking yourself these questions and use your answers as your planning guide. Fill in this checklist and use it to select the right workout. Get creative with what moves and sequences work best for you. Check all that apply.

1. What are the best motivators to keep you in a fitness program?

   ❏ **I am more motivated when I am with a group.** Enroll in a group class or enjoy your water workouts with a friend.

   ❏ **I prefer to be alone.** Devise a routine based on your preferences, needs, and goals, and schedule yourself alone time in the pool on a regular basis.

   ❏ **I like competitive activities.** Consider keeping a fitness journal and track your achieved duration, intensity, and frequency. Build up in each dimension gradually, and challenge yourself to achieve your personal best. Or water walk (hop, kick, etc.) with a competitive friend with whom your speed and level are compatible, and challenge one another to increase your personal bests.

   ❏ **I just want to have fun.** Start with just a few aerobic moves with fun names and then add on gradually to include whatever strikes your fancy, for instance Noodle Moves, Yoga Booty Ballet, Water Kickboxing, or Water Tai Chi. The sky's the limit! Select the kind of activities you have enjoyed in the past or try something new.

   ❏ **I need a routine that is simple and easy to remember.** To keep it simple, warm up with water walking, follow with the stretch sequence, choose several aerobic moves that you find the most fun, or simply water walk (front, back, sideways, and at varying speeds); then cool down with squats and abdominal strengthening, and end with the same stretch sequence you used in your warm-up.

   ❏ **I need a routine that is mentally and physically challenging and in which new things for me to learn are added every few days.** Start with a sequence that meets your current fitness level and familiarity with the aquatic environment. Each week, add new moves by performing the variations explained at the end of most move descriptions, choose a creative selection from chapter 9, Adding Splash to Workouts, or focus on the physical challenges of Power and Plyometric moves in chapter 7, Intensifying Your Workouts.

   ❏ **I need variety to stay motivated.** Once you have mastered a water workout that matches your level of fitness, choose a new area to move into every so often; switching every three to four weeks often works best. Chapter 9, Adding Splash to Workouts, contains a wide range of move types that can keep you changing your routine for years to come.

2. In the past, what kinds of fitness activities have you been successful with or which do you enjoy most?

   ❏ **I really enjoy dancing and am motivated by anything that feels like dancing.** Be sure to include the aerobics moves, performed in the shallow end of the pool, as described in chapter 5, Benefiting From Aerobic Moves, and moves from the Country Line Dancing and Yoga Booty Ballet in chapter 9, Adding Splash to Workouts. Consider joining a water aerobics class, particularly one that uses dance moves.

   ❏ **I like biking.** To enjoy and train for biking, use flotation biking, in the deep end of the pool: Move #32, Bicycle Pump, Move #73, Noodle Sidewinder, and shallow water Pilates Move #104, Diagonal Bicycle Pump.

   ❏ **I enjoy running.** Flotation running can be very challenging and can create the endorphin release and exhilaration often called "the runner's high." Strive for full range of motion; your stride will be slower, but you meet more resistance in water because of the increased viscosity. Another good training exercise is Move #37, Runner's Stride. Add resistance equipment to your feet for both flotation aerobics and Runner's Stride. Incorporate plenty of abdominal and back strengthening moves from chapter 6, Strengthening and Toning, and chapter 9, Adding Splash to Workouts.

   ❏ **I like to hike.** Include Move #18, Mountain Climbing, and Move #31, Floating Mountain Climb. Consider advancing to Move #75, Kickboard Climb.

   ❏ **I like to golf.** Include water walking to enhance your ability to traverse the course. Always include all of the stretches in the stretch sequence and focus especially on chest stretches and back stretches. To strengthen the muscles of the shoulder joint, perform Move #47 Diagonal Front Shoulder Press and other Upper-Body Strengthening and Toning moves. Stretch #12, Midback Stretch, is particularly important for your swing and for back health. For advanced rotational conditioning, perform Pilates Move #101, The Saw. Perform aerobic Move #25, Jump Twist, to maintain and improve torso rotation reflexes. To enhance your game, practice Water Yoga for enhanced flexibility and balance.

   ❏ **I like to play tennis.** Improve your swing and stabilization with Move #45, Sport Training Racket Sweep. If you are an aggressive player, enhance tennis legwork with the Power Squat series, Moves #60 to 65; and Plyometric Moves #66, Peter Pan Side Leap; #67, Hurdle Hop; #20, Mogul Hop; #68, Dolphin Jump; and #71, Hip-Hop Hurray. If you tend more to tame doubles or are engaging in rehabilitative exercise, enhance your footwork with Moves #13, Step Wide Side; #16, Sailor's Jig; #22, Rocking Horse; #21, Knee-Lift Press-Back; and #17, Jump Forward Jump Back. Refine your reflexes with Country Line Dancing Moves #77 to 81. To strengthen the stability of the shoulder joint, perform Move #47 Diagonal Front Shoulder-Press and Move #57 Traffic Cop. Always include all of the stretches in the stretch sequence and focus especially on chest stretches and back stretches. Stretch #12, Midback Stretch, is particularly important for your swing and for back health. For advanced athletic conditioning, challenge your core strength with Pilates Move #101, The Saw. Perform aerobic Move #25, Jump Twist, to enhance rotational reflexes.

❏ **I enjoy martial arts.** You will probably enjoy Water Tai Chi, Moves #82 to 88, which is performed faster in water than on land, and the explosive moves of Water Kickboxing, Moves #89 to 93. These moves can also enhance your speed, agility, and coordination in your land-based martial arts practice.

Set Your Fitness Goals

What kind of fitness goals do you have? Choose up to ten and then rank the top five by prioritizing from numbers 1 to 5, with 1 being the most important, in terms of what you would like to accomplish first and foremost.

I want to:

❏ have more energy. a, b, c, i, k*, l, t

❏ release my tension and frustration. a, c, e, f*, i, k*, m*, t

❏ challenge my cardiovascular system and improve my aerobic endurance. a, b, c, e, i, k*, w*

❏ challenge my cardiovascular system and improve my anaerobic system. b, g, h, i, m*, n, u*

❏ achieve overall body toning. e, g, h, m, t, u*

❏ have better core strength and sleek abdominal muscles. e, g, h, m*, n, q, t, u*

❏ have better upper-body strength. o

❏ tone my hips and thighs. e, g, h, i, p, u*

❏ manage or lose weight. a, g, h, i, l, m*, n, s, v, x

❏ improve my athletic or sport performance. e, g, h, i, k*, m*, n, t, u*, w

❏ be better at running without getting injuries related to impact shock. e, g, h, i, n, p, q, u*, w

❏ enhance my heart health. a, f, j, k*, t

❏ relieve and prevent back pain. r, q, a, c, g, h*, i, j, n, , t*, u*

❏ overcome injuries. g, h*, i, j, n, q, r, t*, u*

❏ create a calmer energy and connect body, mind, and spirit while getting and staying fit. t

❏ feel more flexible, be able to use my joints better, and improve my range of motion. c, g, i, j, q, t, u*

❏ become more stable and be better at avoiding falls. d, e*, f*, g, j, m*, n, q, r, t*, u*

❏ have stronger bones and avoid osteoporosis. a, d, e*, f*, g, m*, q, r, u*

* Within your current fitness capability and only if you are pain-free.

Now you are ready to start thinking about how you are going to accomplish the top five goals you have prioritized.

Find out which actions are most likely to move you toward accomplishing your highest priority goals: Place a tally mark in front of the appropriate letter each time that letter appears next to one of your top five goal responses to the prior question. Circle the letters with the most tally marks. Base your personal workout on those items. Emphasizing the guidelines with the most tally marks takes you closer to your goals. Check out the information next to the rest of the letters with tally marks; each contains information that can enhance your success with your goals. (As with any workout, see your health care professional and discuss your water exercise plan before you begin, especially if you have been sedentary, ill, or injured.)

Build your aerobic endurance by starting at your baseline level (see Your Personal Fitness Profile). Each week, monitor your response. If you feel that you have mastered that level of duration and intensity, increase in either duration *or* intensity by 10 percent. So, if you are water walking 30 minutes, add 3 minutes. To increase intensity, increase your speed or add resistance equipment, but do so gradually.

Use aerobic interval training. Warm up and stretch. Walk for 2 minutes, and then run, fast walk, or hop for 2 minutes. Repeat, alternating between moderate and higher intensity for the entire aerobic sequence, ending with a gradual cool-down and slow aerobic moves such as water walking.

a. Include lots of aerobic moves in shallow, waist- to chest-depth water.

b. Include many hopping moves, but within your current ability to tolerate them without pain or discomfort.

c. Employ plyometric moves.

d. Use squat and squat step moves.

e. Gradually increase your intensity with squats until you can master advanced power moves.

f. Run in the deep end of the pool with flotation. Build your duration gradually, by 10 percent at a time, and include interval training days on which you run fast for several minutes and then run more slowly or stride for several minutes.

g. Select the right moves for your condition from chapter 10, Special Workouts for Special Needs. Include a complete array of stretches and range-of-motion exercises.

h. In your aerobics sequence, build up gradually and cool down gradually; spend plenty of time in the peak aerobics section (increase the intensity gradually over a period of weeks and months).

i. In each aerobics sequence, build intensity gradually and cool down gradually. Focus on maintaining a moderate level of aerobic intensity. Lengthen the duration of your aerobic sequence gradually, over weeks or months, and strive to build up to at least 45 minutes of aerobic activity; Add no more than 10 percent additional minutes at a time, and do so when you have mastered the current level of duration.

j. Include the full array of muscle moves from chapter 6, Strengthening and Toning. Over time, as your fitness level advances, consider adding higher intensity power and plyometric moves from chapter 7, Intensifying Workouts, and Water Kickboxing from chapter 9, Adding Splash to Workouts.

k. Include and focus on "Abdominal Workout Techniques: Abs that Rock," in chapter 6, Strengthening and Toning. Consider including noodle workouts from chapter 9, Adding Splash to Workouts.

l. Include and focus on the upper-body moves in chapter 6, Strengthening and Toning.

m. Include and focus on the lower-body moves in chapter 6, Strengthening and Toning. Consider including power moves from chapter 7, Intensifying Workouts.

n. Include and focus on the moves for posture enhancement in the back and neck, as described in chapter 6, Strengthening and Toning.

o. Follow the workout to relieve and prevent back and neck pain in chapter 10, Special Workouts for Special Needs.

p. Determine which body type you have by checking page 153 in chapter 8, and follow the guidelines described for your type or combination of types.

q. Consider engaging in Water Yoga and Water Tai Chi described in chapter 9, Adding Splash to Workouts..

r. Consider engaging in Water Pilates, described in chapter 9, Adding Splash to Workouts.

s. Monitor your aerobic intensity carefully, using the rate of perceived exertion scale. Strive for moderate intensity, or "fairly light" to "somewhat hard," and work on lengthening your duration gradually over weeks and months.

t. Monitor your aerobic intensity carefully, using the rate of perceived exertion scale. Strive to build toward the "hard" level of intensity, and include a gradual aerobic warm-up and cool-down.

u. See the Tone Up and Lose Weight section in chapter 8, beginning on page 155.

Your Fitness Action Plan for Change

How ready are you to begin your water workouts? Out of the three following choices, which one fits you best? Once you have made your selection, complete the follow-up questions to help you move forward toward your goals.

❏ **I'm thinking about it. I will be ready in about 6 months.** Explore the pros and cons of making water workouts a part of your life. Explore the pros and cons of not fitting in water workouts. Decide which side of the "fence" you are ready to sit on and why.

1. What I like about getting started with water workouts:

2. What I don't like about getting started with water workouts:

❏ **I'm almost ready. I will be ready in about 3 weeks or in the next couple of months.** Write down your barriers or roadblocks and brainstorm some ideas for how you could overcome them.

Barriers   How I could overcome them

1.

2.

3.

4.

❏ **I'm ready to start now!** You are more likely to succeed and to stick with your water workouts if you make a plan based on your personality, preferences, needs, and goals, and if you identify what barriers you expect to face and consider how you can overcome them. Ask yourself this question: How confident, on a scale of 1 to 10, am I that I will succeed with making water workouts a regular part of my life? _____ (enter that number here). Why did I choose that number and not a lower number? (enter your answer here) _____ Why did I choose that number and not a higher number (enter your answer here). _____ Why would have to be different for me to choose a 10? (enter your answer here) _____.

What small steps could you take toward making water workouts a regular part of your lifestyle that would make the most difference right now? List the steps here; one step is enough, and three steps are plenty.

a.

b.

c.

How will you celebrate your successes and reward yourself for sticking to your water workout goals or for making progress?

❏ I will be rewarded by feeling better and having more energy or by performing my sport better.

❏ I will buy myself something nice to enhance my water workouts.

❏ I will take my family out to the beach for a fun outing.

❏ Other: _____

Note: The italicized *f* and *t* following page numbers refer to figures and tables, respectively.

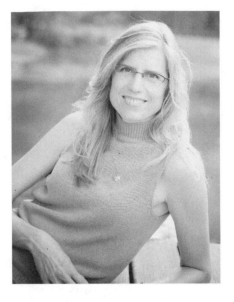

For more than 20 years, **MaryBeth Pappas Baun, MEd**, has been empowering people to make healthy lifestyle changes. A master teacher who has mentored many other instructors and is seen as a fitness guru, she continues to apply those skills in her own practice as a trainer and wellness coach. Her work as a consultant with a mission of developing wellness with others has done just that for the thousands of people who have attended her classes, seminars, and workshops and read her books and articles. Pappas Baun has operated her own wellness and fitness training company since 1982, serving large and small corporations, educational institutions, health care groups, and community organizations. She has also led trainings and wellness programming as a staff employee for Kaiser Permanente, Goodrich Aerospace, and the Cancer Prevention Division at the University of Texas M.D. Anderson Cancer Center.

Pappas Baun is currently a member of the National Wellness Association, the Corporate Health Awareness Team, and the Houston Wellness Association. She has also been a member of the American Council on Exercise (ACE), the American College of Sports Medicine (ACSM), the Aquatic Exercise Association, and the Aerobics and Fitness Association of America (AFAA). She received certifications as a personal fitness trainer in 1995 from the National Academy of Sports Medicine, as an aquatic exercise instructor in 1990 from the Aquatic Exercise Association, as a health and fitness instructor in 1988 from ACSM, and as a group exercise instructor in 1988 from ACE and in 1986 from AFAA. In her leisure time, Pappas Baun enjoys being active through swimming, hiking, biking, and kayaking. She also enjoys dancing, yoga, tai chi, attending live music events, and reading. She is married to William Boyd Baun, who has been a leader in wellness and worksite health and productivity for over 30 years.